Designing the Patient Room

To Eileen and Tessa

"Humanitarianism consists in never sacrificing a human being to a purpose."

Albert Schweitzer

Sylvia Leydecker

De signing the Patient Room

A New
Approach
to Healthcare
Interiors

Birkhäuser
Basel

The publisher and the author wish to thank the following
companies for their participation in this book:

AGROB BUCHTAL
Gira
KALDEWEI
nora systems
wissner-bosserhoff GmbH

Layout, cover design and typesetting
Reinhard Steger, Maria Martí Vigil, Clàudia Serra, Barcelona
www.proxi.me

Project management
Henriette Mueller-Stahl, Berlin

Translation
Julian Reisenberger, Weimar
(except for contribution by Alan Dilani)

Copy editing
Michael Wachholz, Berlin

Production
Katja Jaeger, Berlin

Paper:
Hello Fat Matt 1.1, 135 g/m^2

Lithography
Oriol Rigat, Barcelona

Printing
Offsetdruckerei Grammlich, Pliezhausen

Library of Congress Cataloging-in-Publication data
A CIP catalog record for this book has been applied for at the
Library of Congress.

Bibliographic information published by the German National
Library
The German National Library lists this publication in the
Deutsche Nationalbibliografie; detailed bibliographic data are
available on the Internet at http://dnb.dnb.de.

This publication is also available as an e-book (ISBN PDF
978-3-03821-110-5) and in a German language edition
(ISBN 978-3-03821-492-2).

© 2017 Birkhäuser Verlag GmbH, Basel
P.O. Box 44, 4009 Basel, Switzerland
Part of Walter de Gruyter GmbH, Berlin/Boston

Printed on acid-free paper produced from chlorine-free pulp.
TCF ∞

Printed in Germany

ISBN 978-3-03821-493-9

9 8 7 6 5 4 3 2 1

www.birkhauser.com

Contents

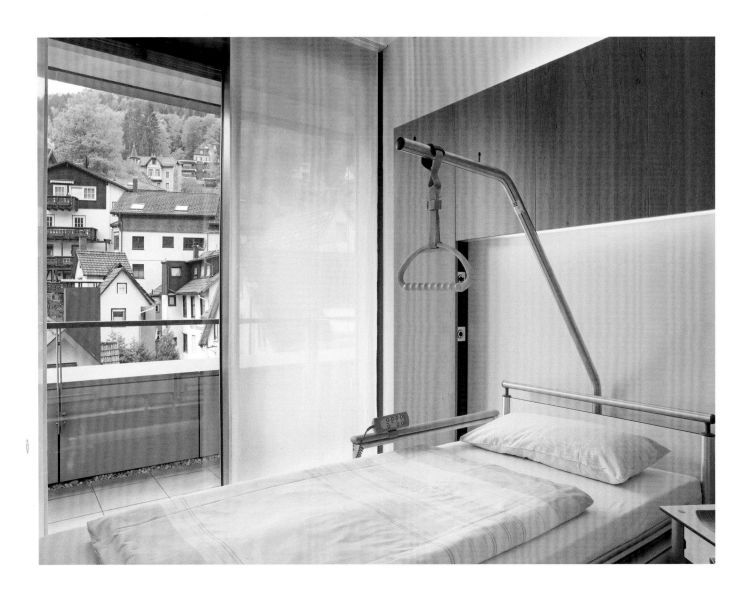

Healing spaces

Fritz von Weizsäcker

Doctor's ward rounds are an important part of daily clinical review activities. As doctors typically visit many patients every day, and ward rounds are only one part of their medical duties, doctors spend a comparatively short amount of time in each patient room. Nursing and care staff spend considerably more time in patient rooms, but they too must divide their time between several rooms. The experience is very different for patients. They leave their room only occasionally, for example for medical tests, surgical procedures or treatments. They find themselves in a room they did not intend to be in, often in a state of anxiety. In the periods between the doctor's visits and treatments, they have ample time to experience the room more intensively than doctors, nurses and care staff. Perfect hygiene – surely a matter of course in this day and age – is just one aspect. Practical requirements are another immediate concern, for example where to place one's clothes and personal belongings, where visitors can sit, how comfortable the bed is and whether the room's door can keep out the noise of hospital activities. Lying in bed, they take in the brightness of the room, the colours of the walls, and study any pictures and decorations for much longer than any of the hospital staff do. All these aspects have a substantial influence on the patients' overall well-being and their impression of the hospital. Immaculate hygiene and a well-designed, usable room reinforces their trust in the clinic, while a pleasant atmosphere lightens their mood. A patient room is, therefore, much more than merely a functional room. Its design requires six eyes: those of the architect, of the hospital staff and, most importantly, of the patient. Successfully bringing these different perspectives into line is what makes a good "healing space".

Fritz von Weizsäcker is an internist and has been Head of the Department of Internal Medicine I at the Schlosspark Klinik in Berlin since 2005.

Introduction

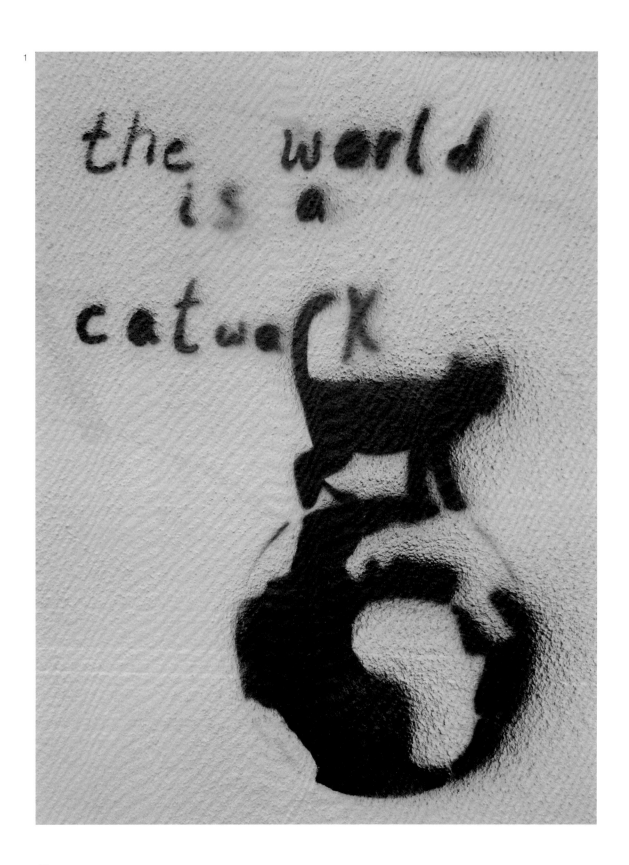

Function versus emotion – "human-centred design"

Hospitals are not only places for treating disease and illness but also institutions for promoting health. This subtle distinction refocusses the perception of hospitals as places of recuperation and healing. The World Health Organisation (WHO) defines health as a balance of factors and needs that contribute to a general sense of well-being. Ups and downs, like periods of stress and relaxation, are a normal part of life. We can weather them as long as they are reasonably balanced. It is when they fall out of balance that we fall ill, and it is here that hospitals come into play. Regardless of whether publicly or privately-operated, whether acute care hospitals, university hospitals, rehabilitation or psychosomatic care clinics, the focus is always on helping individuals in need of help to recover. The common denominator is, regardless of social or cultural background, always the patient's need, level of distress or anxiety. For the patient, a vital remedial factor is a sense of trust, security and emotional reassurance, and the hospital environment can contribute to this. Indeed, it has been shown that architecture and interior architecture can significantly benefit the process of healing, recuperation, or even just the improvement of a condition.

But when it comes to the interior design, it is the financial demands of the healthcare system that dominate: patient care, skilled staff shortages, legislation and subsidies all play a major role in dictating how money is spent. The resulting pressure on available finances inevitably places greater focus on economic efficiency and functionality, on measurable facts, target values, throughput and profit maximisation than on good design and pleasant environments. This is understandable in as far as it addresses the interests of various stakeholders, such as the operators, insurance and management personnel.

But where does this leave the actual person visiting the hospital, the patients and their needs, anxieties and emotions? In today's hospital planning, the patient is more often than not part of a process optimisation system. Patients must fit predefined patterns or else they disrupt the smooth flow of work processes. Patients – each of them diverse individuals – are treated as "standard clinical cases" which can be optimised for profitability. The ongoing unbroken economisation of processes means that patients must be processed as quickly and efficiently as possible through the hospital system. How else can one explain the prioritisation of profitable cases, the rising number of operations or shorter inpatient residence durations for the same fixed charge?

At the same time, one can observe a gradual shift from patient to customer, especially in lucrative sectors and for affluent clients. On the one hand, customers have wishes, expectations and opinions that need to be addressed. On the other, hospitals are increasingly competing with one another for lucrative customers. As such, head doctors want their patients to have comfortable, attractive and well-designed interiors. Nevertheless, the person, the patient, is central to the philosophy, values and mission of every hospital, all over the world. It is a place of physical healing, mental reassurance, safety and security. For the design of hospitals, this means creating a good quality of life through a good-quality environment, especially where patients spend most of their time: in their patient room. It is parameters such as these that serve as quality indicators and ultimately influence the patient's choice of hospital.

There are, of course, natural limits to the desired atmosphere of well-being one can achieve: after all, people rarely feel well when they are ill. Well-being is therefore relative. In this respect, patients share the hospital operators' desire to keep inpatient durations as short as possible. Nevertheless, people, and especially ill people, recover more quickly in environments in which they feel comfortable and at ease.

9

Staff

A people-focussed hospital environment also means designing for the needs of the staff who are on duty 24 hours a day, seven days a week. Medical staff – doctors, nurses and carers – spend a considerable part of their lives in the hospital environment. As such, hospital interiors should help reduce the stress and workload of their demanding job. Interiors that facilitate smooth working processes, provide opportunities for relaxation and are pleasant, attractive and uplifting to work in are also attractive to new staff. People like working in environments in which they feel valued and motivated, and data shows that the incidence of sick leave and staff fluctuation is lower where people enjoy working, resulting in smoother working conditions. Good-quality environments are also an important factor in the competition for skilled staff as they are relevant for job satisfaction.

Economics

As competition for patients and skilled medical staff increases, so too does interest in well-designed hospital interiors. From the client's perspective, interior architects must bring time, professional competency and process-oriented thinking to the design of corresponding hospital spaces. In addition to being able to explain alternatives and describe the respective qualities of materials, they also need to develop a clear rationale that considers the overall need for cost-effective work processes and economisation. The design of interiors influences how staff, patients and visitors behave and interact within them, contributing on the one hand to facilitating work processes and on the other to providing pleasant recovery conditions. Ultimately, well-designed hospital interiors support and reflect the high quality of medical care provision, and as such help raise the profile of the hospital's image.

From Rudolf Virchow and Florence Nightingale to interior architecture

A look into the history books is instructive in understanding how hospital care has evolved. The doctor, pathologist and prehistorian Rudolf Virchow (1821–1902), who practiced for many years at the renowned Charité hospital in Berlin, saw medicine as a social science that should promote public health for everyone, and advocated the combination of medicine and nursing as the best means of helping sick people. But it was Florence Nightingale (1820–1910) in England who established nursing as a true counterpart to medical care and laid the foundation for the modern Western healthcare system. She reformed the system of nursing in the 19th century, professionalising it as a competency in its own right. Her writings are regarded as a cornerstone of modern nursing theory.

The third component, alongside medicine and nursing, is interior architecture as it defines the reciprocal relationship between people and the spaces they occupy. For optimal provision of care for the sick, medicine, healthcare and interior architecture should ideally go hand in hand.

Hotel atmosphere

The design of modern, high-quality patient rooms often attempts to emulate the atmosphere and visual characteristics of a hotel. The associations this evokes are intentional: patients want to (and should) feel as comfortable and well looked-after as possible when recovering from an illness or complaint – in the first instance through medical care, but also through appropriate nursing and care provision to serve the patient's various needs, and, finally, through the atmosphere of the room itself, which should help ease the patient's recovery. In short, given their predicament, patients want to feel as comfortable as possible.

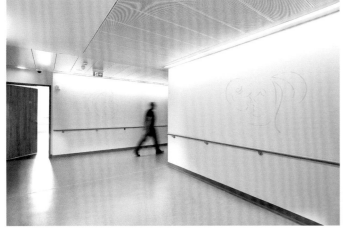

2   Entrance to a patient room in the context of the wayfinding system. 100% interior Sylvia Leydecker, Rems-Murr Hospital, Winnenden, Germany

3   Qualified medical staff are in action 24 hours a day, seven days a week. TAMassociati, Health Centre in a refugee camp, Iraq

4   Hospitals are a part of all cultures and nations of this world.

5   Typical makeshift note in a hospital – no need to be alarmed

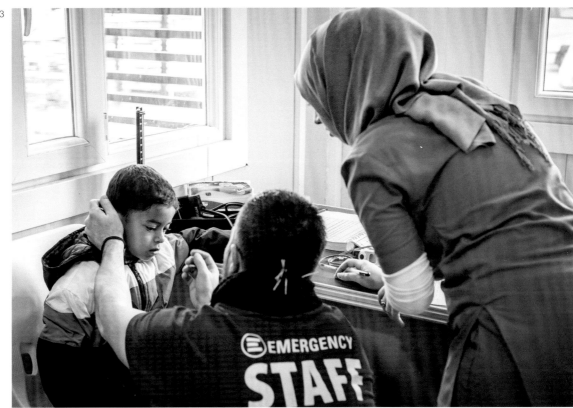

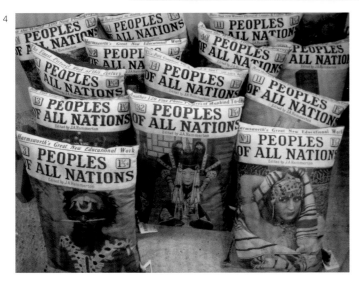

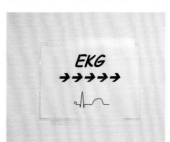

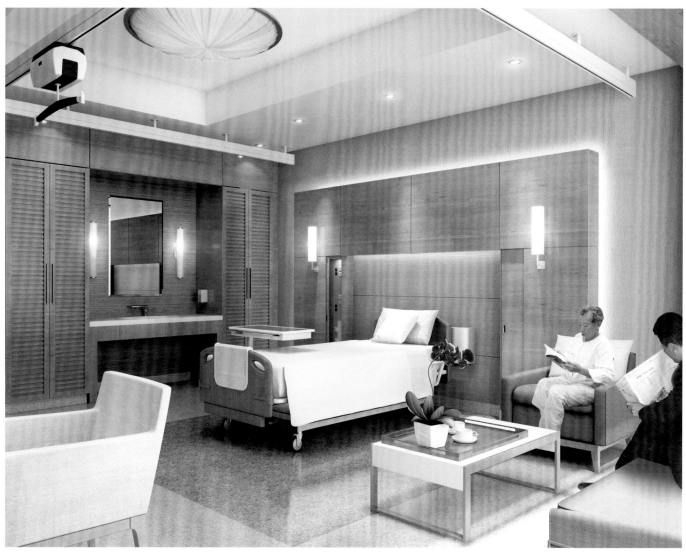

Multi-sensory experiences

Contact to nature and the careful use of colour, light, form, texture, acoustic and haptic qualities all provide additional ways of offering patients rich, multi-sensory experiences that appeal to several senses at once. The multi-sensory effect that environments have, while undeniable, is rarely considered in the design of modern interiors, which concentrate almost exclusively on the visual appearance. That was not always the case. In ancient Baghdad, which was well-known in the Orient for its healing arts, multi-sensory design was already being practised. Baghdad's gardens were reportedly not only beautiful to behold but also planted with fragrant roses, irrigated by bubbling fountains, with cool spots in the shade to sit and enjoy the birdsong – a feast for the senses. Such design principles and the effect they have offer lessons for modern hospital design, where they can help provide patients with pleasant, uplifting surroundings to speed up their recovery. It is hard to imagine how the characterless, utilitarian rooms of many typical modern hospitals can help support the process of recovery.

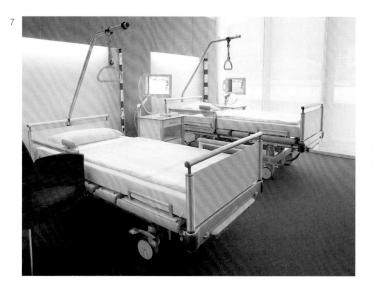

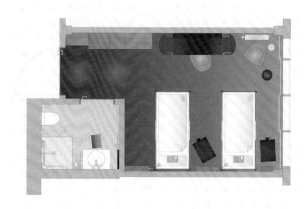

6   High-end hotel atmosphere for affluent patients. CallisonRTKL, Shanghai Changzheng Pudong Hospital, China

7   Corporate interior design with concealed technological equipment for a clinic group. 100% interior Sylvia Leydecker, Sana Clinics, Bad Wildbad, Germany

8   Floor plan of a two-bed patient room variants. Sana Clinics, Bad Wildbad.

9   All design is communication – including the design of spaces. 100% interior Sylvia Leydecker, Sana Clinics Headquarters, Ismaning near Munich, Germany

10 Board lounge of the Sana Clinics Headquarters.

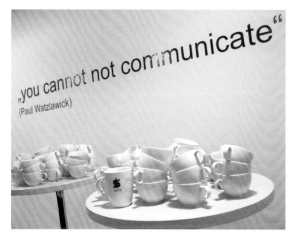

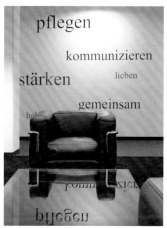

Rooms are complex constructs of multiple factors that we perceive as a multi-sensory experience. Exactly how the perception of healthy people differs from that of sick people is not known, but it is fair to assume that a sick person, depending on their condition, will have an impaired, or at least altered sense of perception – a heightened sensitivity to sound, for example, or the temporary lapse of one or of several senses. Conscious and subconscious perception varies from person to person, whether or not they are sick. The delirium experienced by people exposed to constant noise during intensive care testifies to this.

Interplay of people and space

The interplay of people and space, and how space – the environment – affects people's behaviour, has been known since the time of Charles Darwin. Applied to the design of hospital interiors, this means that rooms and spaces for patients, staff and visitors must be planned meticulously to sensitively incorporate and unify diverse perspectives. In practice, this is typically a balancing act between emotional and functional demands:

13

on the one hand a human-centred approach and the wish to create a pleasant atmosphere, and on the other the demands of process optimisation, hygiene requirements, cost-effectiveness and ecological concerns.

Patient safety

During their stay in hospital, the safety and security of patients is paramount. A central aspect is the prevention of infections spreading in hospitals.

The Hungarian physician Ignaz Semmelweis was the first to present microbiological findings which, despite being widely scorned in the day, prompted the introduction of strict hygiene measures that led to a drastic reduction in childbed fever. Robert Koch and Louis Pasteur later went on to lay the foundations for modern bacteriology and microbiology, after which the need for hygiene earned widespread acceptance. In analogy to Semmelweis, one can therefore assert that the environment can be potentially deadly. If hygiene concerns are ignored in the design of rooms, they can become the cause of infections that may lead to death. This can and must be avoided. Hands are the most common means of transmission, but infections can also be communicated by other means.

While there are many hygiene rules that contribute to patient safety, they are only of value when actively practised and monitored. Patient safety is endangered all too often because other concerns such as work processes and organisation, profit maximisation or even aesthetic concerns, are prioritised. In the design of patient rooms, all these aspects – the functional demands such as process optimisation, safety and hygiene as well as the emotional and aesthetic requirements – need to be reconciled at an affordable price.

Liability prevention also serves as a motor for the development of preventative measures, where design can play a role in improving patient safety.

This applies equally to aspects such as fall prevention measures, which may potentially save hospitals protracted liability litigation, as it does to the prevention of infections through the transmission of nosocomial germs. Consequently, there are many reasons why hospitals cannot be designed like hotels. The challenge when designing a patient room and associated areas is to achieve a symbiosis between the specific patient safety requirements of hospitals and the desire to create an environment that promotes patient well-being.

Healing environments and Evidence-Based Design (EBD)

The effect environments have on people and their emotional well-being has been studied and proven in the fields of Evidence-Based Design and salutogenic design. Both fields are now widely recognised as providing a scientific basis for measuring and demonstrating the beneficial effects of design (over and above the aesthetics) on patients. The concept of "Healing environments" promotes the well-being and healing process of patients by positing an environment that is friendly to patients as well as to staff, and is intelligently organised and human-centred. In the "Healing environment" concept, the patient is the focus of the design of patient rooms. An environment that also caters to the needs of everyone involved in the healing process – doctors, nursing staff and relatives – benefits the overall patient experience.

IT and digitisation

IT and digitisation have made significant inroads into the fields of medicine and healthcare and are increasingly becoming an integral part of room designs. Current concept designs for patient rooms

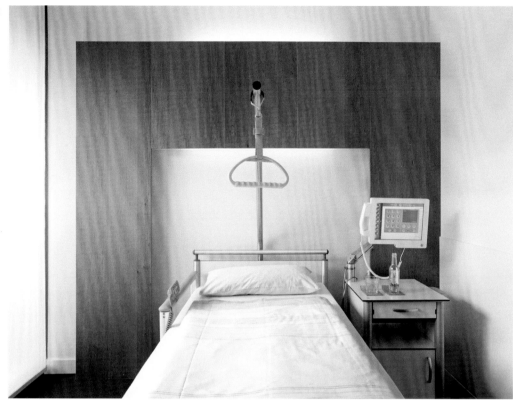

11 The warm surfaces of the wood panelling, a cutout for the bed, and concealed supply lines and technology help create an atmosphere of comfort and trust far removed from typical sterile hospital interiors. 100% interior Sylvia Leydecker, Sana Clinics, Bad Wildbad, Germany

12 Functional details can be accessed and concealed as needed. NXT Health in collaboration with Evans & Paul and Dolan & Traynor; DuPont™ Corian®, Patient Room 2020 Prototype, New York, USA

13 The consistent use of white communicates a sense of cleanliness. Stöbe Architekten, Alfried Krupp Hospital, Essen, Germany

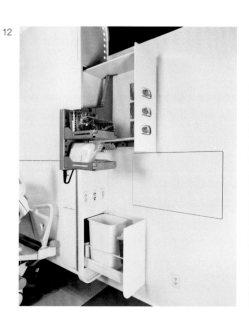

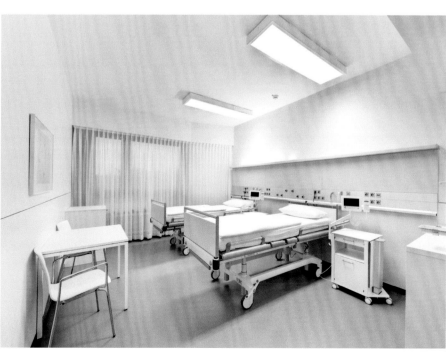

of the future offer an ambitious glimpse of future possibilities, although often paired with a futuristic look: smart, digital and sterile, with streamlined shapes, white, shiny surfaces accentuated with glittery asteroid-like silver trim, and futuristic digital surfaces; in short, rather cool and impersonal. Sensors alert staff when action needs to be taken, procedures are optimised for maximum efficiency and minimum intrusion, and processes are optimised based on patient data. The communication methods of the upcoming generations Y and Z differ markedly from those of generation X and will, no doubt, affect how we relate to IT in future. While organic-amorphous designs in a Star Wars look are not necessarily the answer, an appropriate language for integrating digital content into room design will need to be found that is digital, smart and sustainable.

Almost all perspectives and visions for the patient room of tomorrow portray spatial scenarios for smart, progressive medical care in which, since the beginning of the millennium, IT plays an increasing role in addressing the problems we face. But faith in technology alone – sensors, microsystems and lighting controls – does not hold the answer. Equally important is the creation of environments and atmospheres that promote the overall well-being, recovery and healing process of patients. Future patient rooms and accompanying spaces must therefore be more than purely functional, sterile spaces; they must be designed as spaces of well-being. Sensors that allow lighting scenarios to be changed interactively, that adjust room temperature or soundscapes are potentially useful applications if applied to positively influence the atmosphere of the room and improve the emotional state of the patient. The future lies in hybrid spaces in which analogue and digital experiences blend into a single reality – not an Augmented Reality for the eyes and ears alone as provided by AR-goggles, but a true integration of reality and technology that also involves other senses.

Smart nanomaterials

Healthy building means making the best of both traditional and smart materials. On the one hand, it is imperative in an environmentally-responsible age to employ sustainable, certified products and building materials, energy-efficient light sources and resource-efficient systems. On the other, self-cleaning surfaces that reduce cleaning costs and anti-bacterial surfaces that improve hygiene should also be considered, as should the possibility of saving energy using Phase Change Materials (PCMs) or high-efficiency insulation systems such as Vacuum Insulated Panels (VIPs). Electrochromic glazing can obviate the need for other mechanical solar shading systems and high-efficiency photovoltaic (PV) modules can produce energy in-house. Better illumination can be achieved not only by maximising natural light but also by using interactive, energy-efficient LEDs and OLEDs. Ultra-high performance concrete (UHPC) makes it possible to construct more slender constructions, and lightweight but strong materials such as carbon have revolutionised product design. In future, high-tech medical care will go hand-in-hand with high-tech hospital interiors that need not necessarily emulate the streamlined Star Wars-inspired interiors and amorphous white mineral composite materials that to date have dominated futuristic design concepts.

The days of particle board, carpets, curtains and wallpaper, as used almost universally today, are numbered. In future, carbon and foils will play an increasingly important role in the design of products and building interiors. Innovations such as 3D printing, and attributes such as ultra-lightweight, strong, self-cleaning, translucent, transparent, conductive, luminous, electrochromic, energy-retentive and the like offer inspiring possibilities for future hospital design. Furniture and fittings – cupboards, beds and bedside tables – will then no longer be made of particle board but of ultra-lightweight, self-cleaning materials. Walls will be switchable from opaque to translucent, and lighting foils will enable new versatile approaches to designing and controlling illumination.

Interior design as part of the architecture

The architecture of a building, whether a new, existing or even historic listed building, serves as a framework for the design of interiors and patient rooms. Hospitals differ greatly in size and scale, from small, compact and medium-sized facilities, to conglomerates of different clinics built at different times on a single extensive site, to vast mega-structures such as university hospitals. These are the contexts into which private healthcare patient rooms or premium wards will be inserted.

Hospitals are, by definition, highly complex facilities with comparatively complicated functional areas that need to respond flexibly to the respective demands. Once built, it is rare for hospitals to undergo significant alterations. Nevertheless, they need to be built to adapt flexibly to changing use patterns and room divisions. Generous floor spaces are a good way of ensuring flexibility and adaptability in future. However, the dictate of space optimisation typically runs counter to this, resulting in the creation of individual optimised rooms of minimal size. Interior architecture needs to work within these parameters to make the best of the given situation.

In ideal circumstances, the architecture of the interior should support and transport the intentions and parameters of the overall architectural concept for the building, including its relationship to the site and location, and not least the concept and identity of the respective hospital. It should respect and enhance the overall design, meshing with its architectural surroundings to create a coherent architectural experience. The choice of materials and palette of colours, the views inside and out, the proportions of the spaces are, for example, all relevant parameters for a coherent dialogue between

14 Digital networking is the primary topic of the "FutureCare" section of the CeBIT trade fair. 100% interior Sylvia Leydecker, FutureCare 2010, CeBIT Hanover, Germany

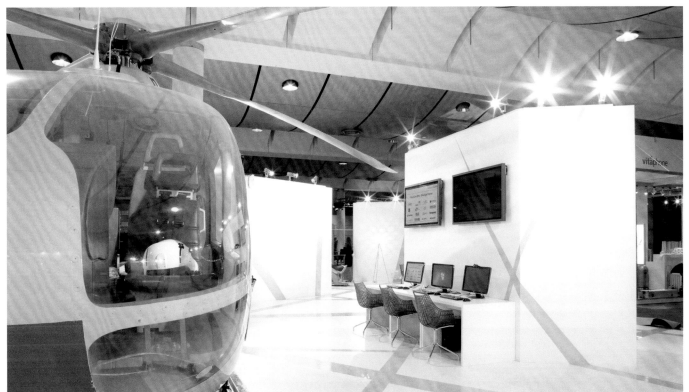

14

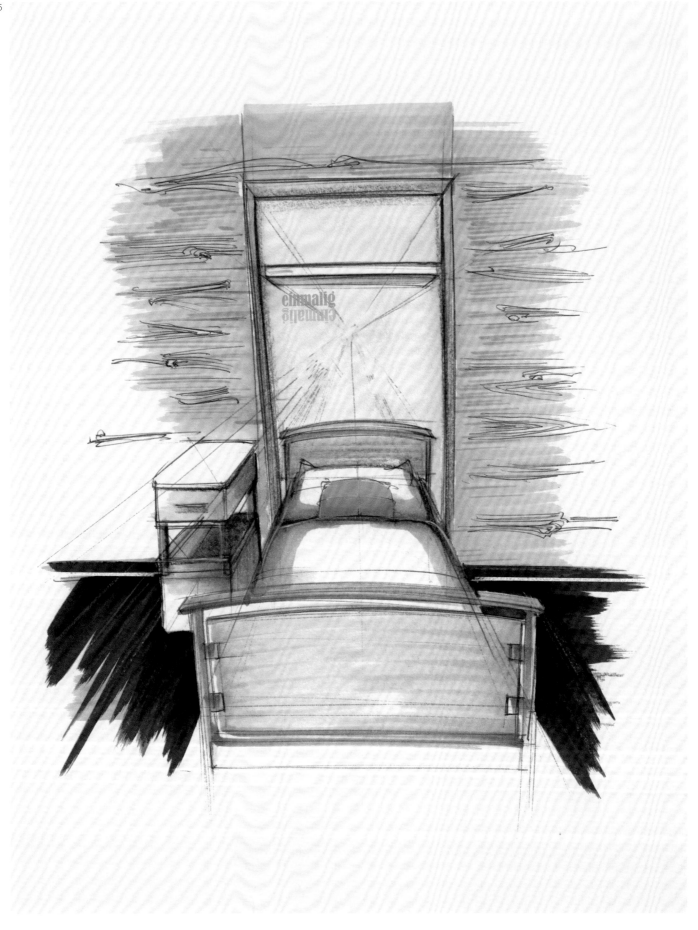

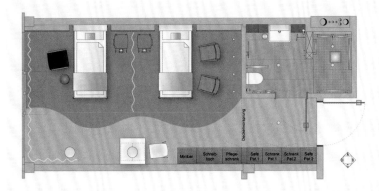

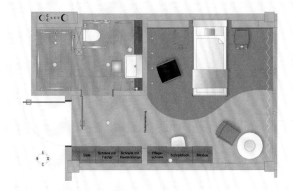

15 Every person and every patient is unique.
100% interior Sylvia Leydecker, Rems-Murr Hospital,
Winnenden, Germany

16 The wavy floor pattern marks the different parts
of this two-bed room and defines areas of greater
privacy. 100% interior Sylvia Leydecker, St. Vinzenz
Hospital, Düsseldorf, Germany

17 The design of the floor covering defines the different
parts of this single-bed patient room. St. Vinzenz
Hospital

the architectural design of the interior and the building as a whole. The interior architecture also relates to the wider built environment. The interiors define, for example, the façade of a building where they are visible from outside or when illuminated at night. They may open onto their surroundings or be inwardly oriented. The design of interiors must therefore also respond to the respective urban or rural environment. As such, interior architects must consider not just the design of an individual room type but the overall system of the building and its interior.

Interior architecture as an independent design task

The architectural design of hospital interiors is often either a rather rapid affair – shortly before the hospital opens – or an extremely lengthy process. In either case, the process requires that participants and specialists from different disci-plines work together in a team. Professional competency and emotional intelligence are required in equal measure, along with the ability to adapt to and work together with different people and changing constellations with a view to finding constructive solutions.

In ideal cases, the work of interior architects is regarded as an important and indispensable part of the overall design process. Clients must recognise the value of good and healthy interior design for the quality of the patient's hospital experience, as well as the contribution it makes to optimising work processes and accounting, as the resulting economic benefits can be potentially quite considerable. Functional criteria are extremely important in hospital design, sometimes even life-saving. Hygiene is in this context a key aspect of the architectural design, as is wayfinding and the choice of suitable construction methods. The particular challenge when designing hospital interiors is to find a smart balance between functional considerations and addressing the emotional needs of the users.

Single and shared rooms – an international comparison

The typical room for patients with private health insurance is a single room. Patients can control conditions according to their own needs: they can receive visitors, open the window, draw the curtains, change the lighting or switch on infotainment media when they wish. Most of all, a single room ensures privacy and peace and quiet, which is conducive to rest and recuperation. There are none of the disturbances of multi-bed patient rooms, such as unfamiliar sounds, smells, conversations or visitors for other people. A further advantage is the reduced risk of infection from other people. The downside is the risk of loneliness, especially when in hospital for long periods.

Multi-bed patient rooms represent both a positive and negative counterpart to the single room. The company of others is, without doubt, an additional stress factor for patients, for example intrusive coughing and snoring can impact on one's ability to sleep properly. Unfamiliar smells and the reduced sense of privacy are likewise negative characteristics. The risk of infection, either through airborne transmission or through sharing the bathroom and toilet is also higher in rooms with multiple occupants. A positive aspect, by contrast, is the company and social contact in a multi-bed patient room, and improved patient safety as patients can watch out for one another.

In Denmark, single-bed rooms are standard, but in some developing countries around the world, for example in Africa, multi-bed patient rooms are already a comparative luxury. In the USA, the trend is moving towards smaller rooms, while in Germany, rooms are already planned to comparatively tight space constraints, whereby room sizes differ depending on the level of health insurance services. Patients with private health insurance who opt to have a room of their own will receive a more comfortable and better-quality room than patients with regular national health insurance. In other parts of Europe, for example in Vienna, one can still find multi-bed patient rooms for as many as ten people, as "private rooms" are viewed socially as unacceptable and are therefore difficult to implement politically. In Arab countries, by contrast, high-end "royal suites" and "Very-VIP rooms" exist for the ruling families and provide facilities that others patients can only dream of.

18

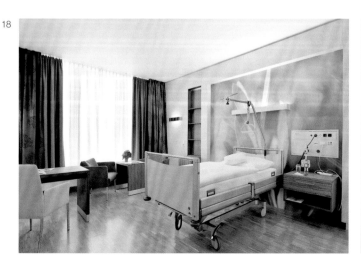

19

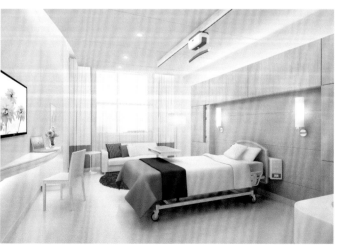

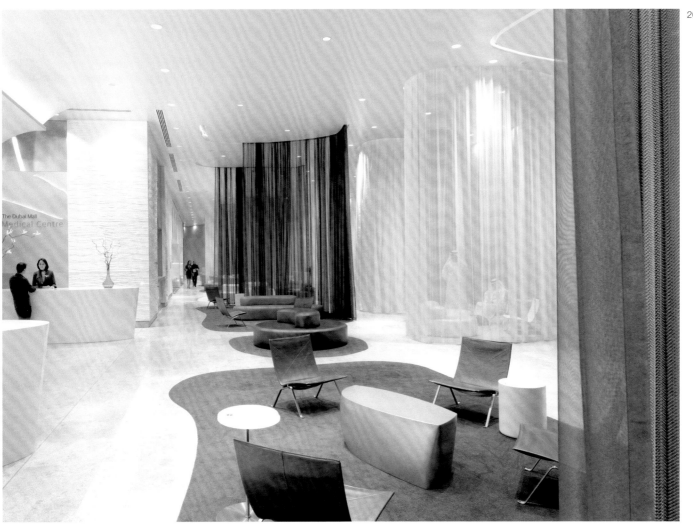

18 A high-class hotel atmosphere
    in a patient room. Brandherm +
    Krumrey, Main-Taunus Private
    Clinic, Bad Soden, Germany

19 High-quality materials and lighting
    systems create a more homely patient
    room. CallisonRTKL, Shanghai Chang-
    zheng Pudong Hospital, China

20 Contrasting floor coverings and
    translucent curtains demarcate separate
    areas. NBBJ, Dubai Mall Medical Center,
    United Arab Emirates

Patient rooms in private clinics – for example in parts of Asia such as Bangkok or Singapore – are typically designed for a more affluent clientele and frequently correspond to the standard of a high-end hotel. Elite, high-price VIP clinics, such as Lenox Hill in the USA, have made headlines through the likes of stars such as Jay-Z and Beyoncé. Paradoxically, the hospitals that clamour for public subsidies and advocate people-centred medical care are also often those that boast such elite VIP wards. This is a dilemma in as much that the paying, privately-insured patients subsidise the regular wards. Nevertheless, the emergence of a two-tier society in healthcare and the resulting social divide are hardly reconcilable with the notion of "putting people first".

Social tensions

The balancing act between "putting people first" and financing this promise remains a difficult global political and social issue. People of all social and cultural backgrounds should be entitled to receive adequate healthcare, and politicians are called on to provide the corresponding means by which this can be realised. After all, they receive their mandate from the people – at least in the democratic nations of this world. The difficulty of reconciling benevolent, charitable principles with the need to find suitably solvent paying patients is a problem that is not new, having first arisen two centuries ago. The extremely unequal distribution of wealth is socially highly contentious and a danger for the health service of potentially significant proportions. In Europe and elsewhere economic migration and swelling numbers of refugees have recently exacerbated the situation. In the USA, the historic healthcare reform of the Obama administration of 2010, which made health insurance available to millions of previously uninsured citizens, may soon be repealed, leaving those who have profited from the reform to an uncertain fate. Morally, every person needs care and protection regardless of their background. A purely technocratic approach would seem to be just as inappropriate and lacking

in humanity as the economisation of the much-vaunted principle of "putting people first". Many medical luminaries and rainmakers have tried and failed when faced with the constraints of this structural problem.

Outlook

The designs shown in this book for patient rooms and their associated areas around the world have one thing in common: the desire to improve patient care through the design of environments that promote their well-being. Inevitably this starts with patients with private health insurance, despite the different structural conditions for healthcare provision around the world. To avoid concentrating solely on elite healing environments for the well-heeled, this book also includes inspiring and very humane projects that are not directly related to the design of patient rooms in hospitals. For example, the Maggie's Centres in England, conceived as drop-in day care centres providing practical, emotional and social support for cancer patients, or the Salam Centre for Cardiac Surgery in Sudan that provides free heart treatment for children and adults alike. Projects from all over the world – from Germany to the USA and Africa, as well as Kuwait, Thailand and China – show a spectrum of different patient room environments. Irrespective of the examples shown in this book, one can expect to see advances in IT, the digital revolution, and modern materials drive the future design of patient rooms – ideally with a human-centred and patient-friendly focus for the benefit of everyone.

21 Coloured walls, floors and glazing sections turn a simple corridor into a kaleidoscope of colour. EwingCole, Children's Hospital of Philadelphia, USA

22 Wayfinding systems help people navigate complex hospital structures. büro uebele visuelle kommunikation, Offenbach Clinic, Germany

23 Patients and staff on the move are an essential part of the process of "hospital treatment". Offenbach Clinic

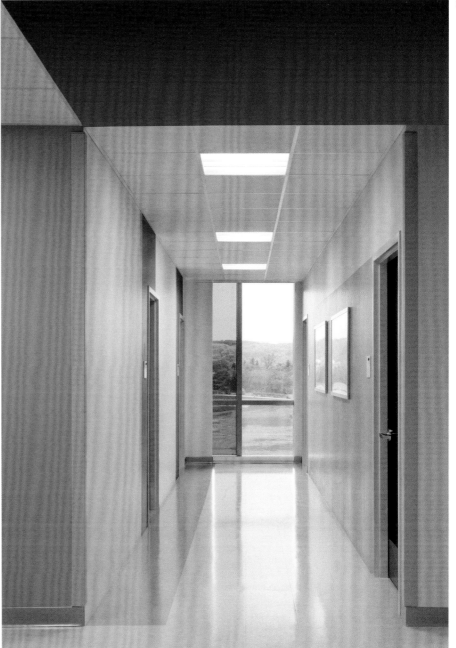

21

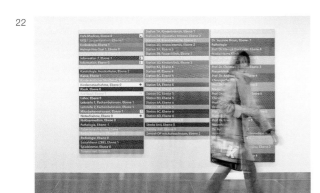

22

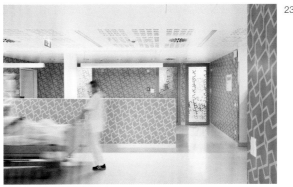

23

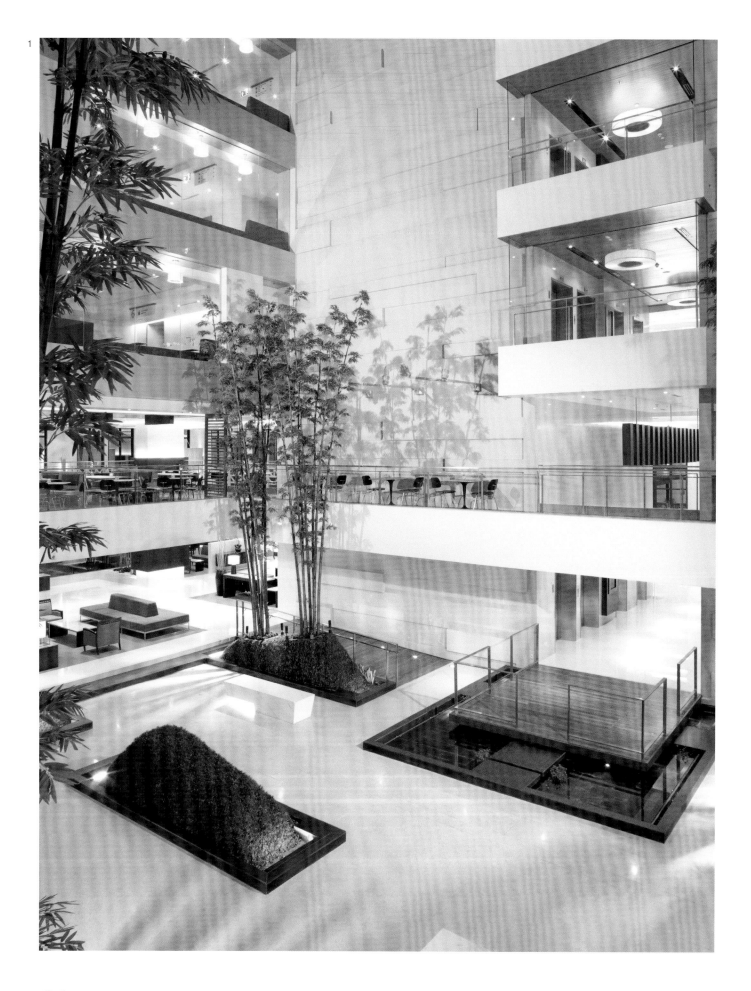

Functional areas

The patient room as primary experience

For patients, the patient room is of central importance as it is here that they spend most time.
The quality of their experience depends on
whether the room merely accommodates their
enforced stay or provides a living environment that
conveys a feeling of trust, safety and well-being
that aids the process of recovery. As such, this
room is often the single most important reason
why a patient decides to choose one hospital over
another. Rooms for patients with private health
insurance are typically better situated, for example on upper levels with a particularly good
view. In addition, corridors, lounges, nursing
stations, reception and waiting areas must also
be considered as part of the interior architecture.

Well-designed patient rooms are environments in
which patients feel comfortable and looked after,
so that they can recover at ease. Impersonal,
utilitarian spaces are entirely inappropriate as they
disregard the emotional qualities that contribute
to patient recovery. A patient room functions first
and foremost as a place of healing, but it is also a
work place, and an economic unit for accounting
purposes. The design of patient rooms can be
vital for optimising work patterns and services,
and therefore for revenue optimisation. Finally, its
atmosphere and aesthetics must correspond to the
class of the institution and give the patient a sense
of being safe and in good hands to enable them to
recover in relaxed, stress-free surroundings.

For patients, the room they occupy is without
doubt their primary experience of a hospital and
therefore a vital component of the interior design.

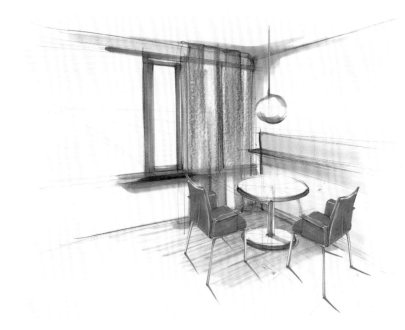

2 Sketch of a dining area in a patient room. 100% interior Sylvia Leydecker, Rems-Murr Hospital, Winnenden, Germany

3 Living area in a patient suite. Jim Clemes, Mother & Child Centre, Luxembourg

4 A two-bed room with two sets of supply lines. Jim Clemes, Mother & Child Centre, Luxembourg

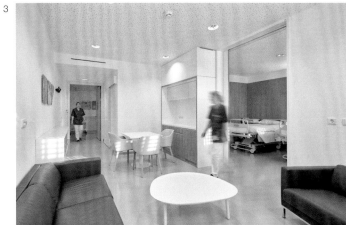

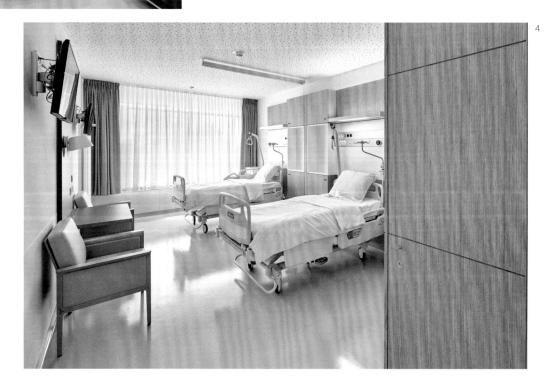

While the basic elements of a patient room seem at first glance straightforward, the need to reconcile the many considerations and requirements in a functioning overall concept is a considerably more complex task. And because the room ultimately serves as a prototype for numerous patient rooms, it is worth investing due care and attention in optimising its design. The consequences of sub-optimal design decisions quickly multiply and can, in the worst case, lead to years of recurring unnecessary friction and wastage in hospital operations. Meticulous planning can therefore save considerable unnecessary costs.

Single-bed versus two-bed rooms

For patients with private health insurance, single-bed rooms are the norm. In Denmark, all new hospital buildings contain only single-bed rooms. In Germany, by contrast, two-bed rooms are commonly provided as a supplementary service option. Each room must therefore be designed for two beds with two sets of supply connections, even if it is used at times as a single room. The second bed is then simply removed or placed out of the way. Depending on occupancy levels, this may be the rule or the exception.

A single room is generally considered to be superior: it offers greater personal privacy, patients have more control over their environment, fewer disturbances and a lower risk of infection from others. Two-bed rooms, on the other hand, offer the possibility of social interaction and better patient safety, because patients effectively "monitor" one another. Older patients in particular often find single rooms isolating. Which variant is better is a topic of ongoing discussion. Other important factors include the size of the room, the proximity to the nursing station and the flexibility of their design. Patients and nurses do not always have the same priorities and which room people end up in often depends on who is choosing: the patient or the nursing staff.

Ultimately, the level of occupancy and the combination possibilities with other patients often determine how rooms are allocated. In two-bed rooms it is necessary to provide two sets of everything and to make it clear which facilities belong to which bed to avoid squabbles over which hook belongs to whom, or people using the wrong towels. In either case, comfort and the atmosphere of the room are primary aspects of the design of both single- and two-bed rooms.

Floor plan

Floor plans of individual patient rooms are typically designed to maximise the efficient use of space with little free space or space for placing items. Luxurious patient rooms are often much more spacious, but should not be too large to avoid the sensation of "horror vacui". In either case, beds should be placed so that they can be reached from three sides, so staff have direct access, especially in the case of an emergency. Medical and nursing staff should be able to see the patient from the door to assess the momentary situation on entering the room. Placing the long sides of beds against a wall can be problematic for patients with restricted motion, for example if they are only able to face or move in one direction. From the patient's perspective, the placement of the bed should permit them to look outside onto greenery, to see people entering via the door, to watch over their belongings in the bedside cabinet and cupboard, and to watch TV.

Freestanding items of furniture and built-in fittings must be incorporated so that they do not obstruct work patterns within the room and provide sufficient space to move around. Fold-down tables are a typical example: they must be large enough to support a food tray but designed with bevelled edges so that they can be fixed to the wall. While these are not always the most aesthetic solution, the need for sufficient space to eat despite the minimal floor plan, or to roll beds out of the room necessitates such special designs for hospitals. In addition, they can

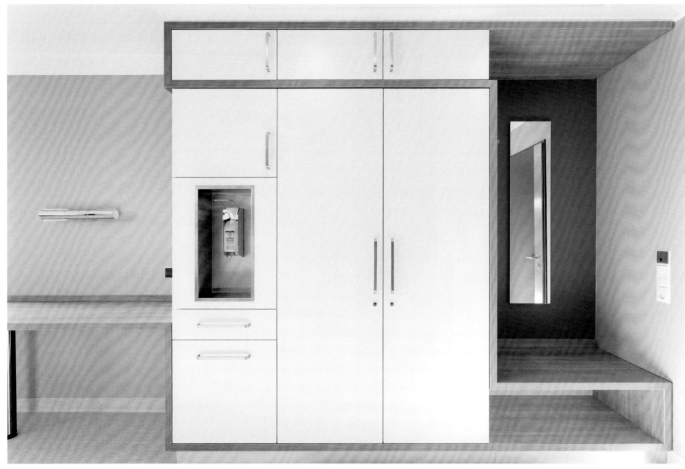

5 A made-to-measure all-in-one unit combines several functions in one. GSP Gerlach Schneider Partner Architekten, Amrum comfort ward, Bremen-Nord Clinic, Germany

provide space for storing personal utensils, newspapers, glasses cases, boxes and so on.

The bed

The bed (with the patient lying in it) is the focal point of a patient room. Compared with hotel beds, hospital beds are veritable "lying machines". The shorter the patient's stay, the more intensively they will be used. Equipped with a range of functions, beds are typically chosen by the nursing management. In terms of aesthetics, choice is limited. Very often only the headboard and foot-board inserts can be chosen to match the room design. In most cases these are high-pressure laminate (HPL) panels available from the manufacturer in a range of standard colours and special designs. The choice varies typically between solid colours and wood-finish effects, popular in private healthcare rooms. Panels with patterns or ornamentation are rarely available. Most hospital beds also provide connections or ports for electronic and electrical equipment, for example TV screens, controls and monitoring devices. Given the speed of advances in digital technology, these may need replacing before the bed itself. Sensors also provide an additional means of adjusting various control and comfort aspects of the bed.

Bed linen

Bed linen plays a major role in defining the visual appearance of hospital interiors. Hospital bedding is by its very nature a potential carrier of bacteria as it is in direct contact with patients. It must therefore be robust enough to withstand repeated rigorous disinfection in the hospital laundry and fit in with hospital logistics. Ideally the bedding should be chosen as part of the room design, rather than the room design having to work around poorly chosen pieces of bed linen to avoid them standing out. Good-quality bed linen, a small-format pillow and a decorative blanket or throw immediately evoke associations with a hotel, and should be favoured over cheap mass-produced wares.

Beds for relatives to stay with their loved ones are also highly appreciated, so that patients can enjoy familiar company.

Rolling beds

Whether beds for regular patients or those for patients paying for supplementary services should be the same or different depends on whether premium patients should be identifiable while "on the move" in the rest of the hospital. Beds must be able to pass through all doors and openings and around corners. The design of rooms must take into account that the travel width of the bed is wider than the bed itself so that bags hung from the bed or arms hanging out of the bed cannot snag on obstacles. Beds can cause significant damage to walls, especially at critical points such as narrow sections and curved stretches, or when moving at speed in urgent situations. Wall protection strips and corner guards are recommended at key points inside and outside the patient room.

The pathways and day-to-day movements of patients and staff should be studied carefully to optimise planning. Carpets, for example, have a higher rolling resistance and require more effort for staff to push. Optimising such aspects can bring time savings in the work processes. Patients, on the other hand, prefer flooring materials and fittings that make spaces more comfortable.

Storage space

A bedside cabinet provides storage directly next to the bed, allowing patients to stow personal belongings within easy reach. Wardrobes, by contrast, can be further away and don't necessarily have to be in sight. Lockable wardrobes help prevent incidences of theft, but bear the risk that the key may get lost. Valuables are often placed in a safe, frequently located within fitted wardrobes. Some hospitals also provide a refrigerator or minibar, either in the cupboard, in a separate item of furniture or within comfortable reach in the bedside cabinet.

Cupboards in patient rooms should be fitted and extend right up to the ceiling, making it unnecessary to clean on top of them. They provide storage for the patient's clothes and sometimes also for their luggage, a minibar, safe and so on. The number and size of compartments, clothes rails and robust coat hangers (which can be branded) is relevant in such cases, as is the choice of suitable fittings with respect to their form, material and surface finish. Better quality fittings are generally more robust, minimising the need for expensive repairs at a later date. A particular problem is the placement and arrangement of storage that can be accessed by wheelchair users. Barrier-free access for patients in wheelchairs should be provided as far as is possible. Storage space for care staff is helpful to allow staff to store corresponding utensils. Likewise, disinfectant dispensers must be provided and can be integrated into furniture and fittings. A wardrobe with mirror provides a place for hanging clothes as well as visitors' coats and jackets.

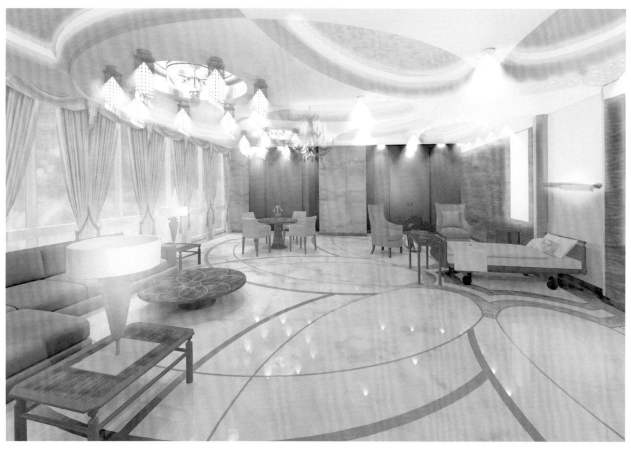

Equipment and fittings – chairs and tables

Comfortable chairs, armchairs and sofas are commonly found in private healthcare patient rooms to provide better comfort. A dining table should offer space for up to two people to eat at once, taking into account the size of the hospital food trays. In premium patient rooms, an armchair with reading lamp is standard, but a seating combination can be desirable, for example for when the extended family comes to visit, as is common in Arab cultures. Upholstery fabrics should be resistant to urine, and stains show less against patterned fabrics. All fabrics and textiles should be robust enough to withstand disinfecting agents. There is no set rule for the height of backrests

and armrests and each option has its respective advantages and disadvantages. High back rests are comfortable but also less hygienic and more susceptible to soiling as the patient's head rests on them (for example with unwashed hair). Chairs without a high back rest will typically last longer. Chairs without armrests are more slender and take up less space, but are also more difficult to get up from. A further problem when lots of visitors arrive at once is that half the family sits on the bed. This can only be avoided in larger suites. In circumstances where this is not the case, the lack of sufficient seating generally means that such visits will continually cause disruption and unacceptable hygienic soiling. At the same time large family visits have a certain charm. A desk with another chair – but not a swivel office chair – can also be advisable in patient rooms.

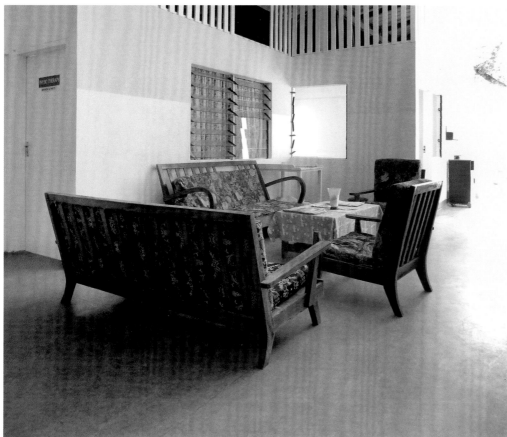

6 Design for a luxurious high-end room for a royal patient. 100% interior Sylvia Leydecker, Jaber Al Ahmad Al Jaber Al Sabah Hospital, Kuwait

7 Where the climate allows: a comfortable open-air waiting area in a hospital in the tropics

8 Private waiting area at a reception area with changing light installation. 100% interior Sylvia Leydecker, Rems-Murr Hospital, Schorndorf, Germany

9 A single unit incorporates a cupboard, wardrobe and suitcase shelf. Oliver Faber Innenarchitektur, comfort ward, JosefCarrée, Bochum, Germany

8

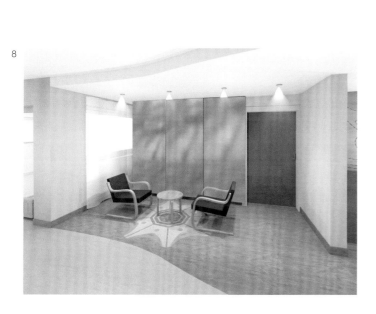

9

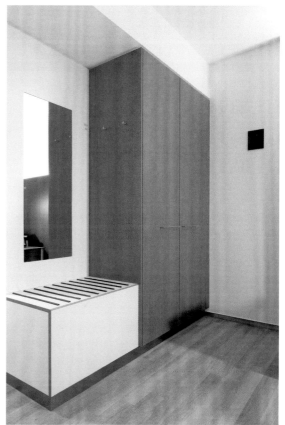

10 A clear, unfussy entry situation.
GSP Gerlach Schneider Part-
ner Architekten, comfort ward,
Ammerland Clinic, Westerstede,
Germany

11 Two washbasins and ample space
for toiletries. GSP Gerlach Schneider Partner Architekten, Amrum
comfort ward, Bremen-Nord
Clinic, Germany

12 A WC with fold-down supports on
both sides, Amrum comfort ward

13 The transparent glass shower
enclosure makes the room feel
larger, Amrum comfort ward

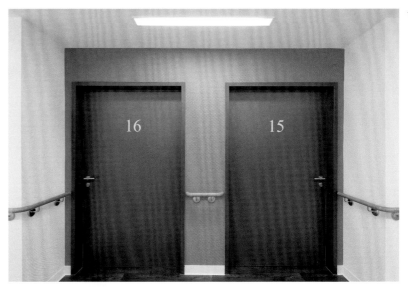

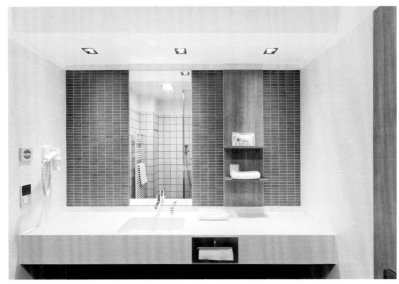

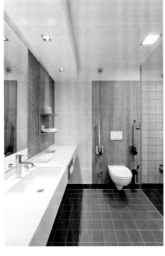

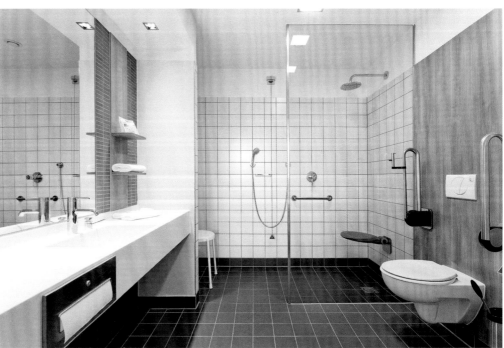

Bathroom

Good hospital bathroom design begins by dispensing with the idea of the "wet cell". Bathrooms in standard patient rooms in Germany are less than 4 m², and only larger in better-class rooms. All necessary fittings and equipment must be incorporated within this limited space, requiring careful planning. The arrangement of a floor-flush shower, the WC and a wheelchair-accessible washbasin needs to be carefully thought out. Grips and handrails should be provided to assist infirm patients but should not look overtly like special aids. Further bathroom fittings include a large mirror, good lighting, sufficient storage space, a hairdryer, shaving mirror, presentable towels and toiletries, and a heated towel rail. Large-format tiles are advisable, not only because of the quality they convey but also because they have fewer joints, which is more hygienic. With anti-slip floor surfaces, a balance needs to be found between providing a firm footing and ensuring hygienic cleaning.

Further fittings and conveniences

Health insurance providers stipulate a range of further fittings and features that are part of their supplementary service packages and can conveniently be billed by hospitals, should they want to provide for these extras. They can range from comfortable, upholstered chairs to adjustable lighting systems that can switch between atmospheric background lighting, light for reading and bright light for medical examinations. Wireless internet access, music, a TV screen for entertainment, as well as working from hospital, are likewise often included in health insurance packages. Far-sighted hospital operators may offer their patients additional complimentary amenities as per their house philosophy, for example flowers, fresh fruit, bathroom cosmetics, a bathrobe and slippers, and so on.

Blinds, shades and privacy curtains

Curtains, and textiles in general, contribute a homely atmosphere to patient rooms. Most curtains, however, are not suitable for use in health-care environments as they can only be washed at low temperatures and cannot be disinfected. Lightweight semi-transparent curtains are usually sufficient to provide a measure of privacy, but to darken a room, a suitably opaque material is required. Ideally, blinds and shades can be regulated electrically from the patient's bed.

Accessibility

Incorporating accessibility means practicing Universal Design: design that can be used by everyone with or without physical disabilities. This means not just wheelchair users but also people with sight or hearing impairments, or even young couples with a pushchair. Barrier-free access to all floors for wheelchair users, disabled toilets, adequate space for movement and high-contrast, legible signage for the poor-sighted improve accessibility in the public areas of hospitals. In patient rooms, this can only be achieved to a limited degree: for example, small bathrooms (such as the 4 m² standard bathroom in Germany) cannot properly accommodate the turning radius of wheelchairs. Floor-flush shower trays or tiled floors, wheelchair-accessible washbasins and mirrors that can be seen from different heights are just some of the possible measures. Handles and buttons that are easy to use and provide predictable haptic responses aid in using equipment. Desks in reception areas and nursing stations should have unobstructed lower-height sections for interacting with wheelchair users. In addition, the layout of the floor plan should set aside space for parking and storing wheelchairs, prams and pushchairs.

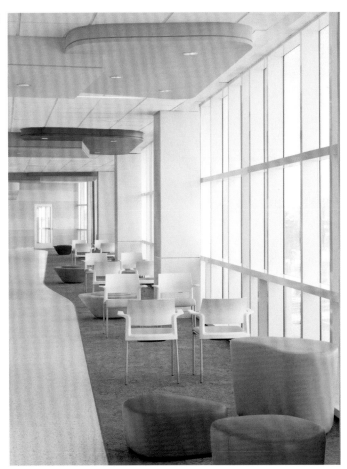
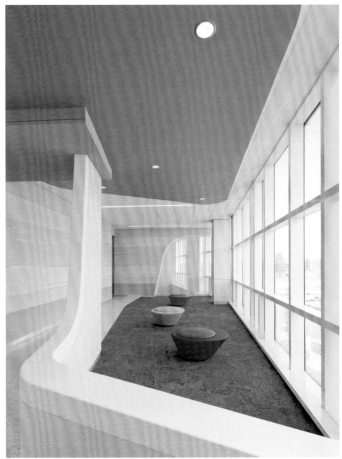

Corridors

Uninspiring, boring, sterile and anxiety-inducing hospital corridors are gradually giving way to light-filled, spacious public circulation spaces with a much more uplifting atmosphere.

Corridors serve primarily as a means of connecting different spaces. They have their own system of wayfinding cues that indicate where one is and where one is going. Corridors often mark transitions into other worlds and are all too often neglected, despite playing an important role in communicating the atmosphere of a hospital. A pleasant atmosphere that exudes tranquillity is ideal for most journeys. Corridors are typically straight with doors on one or both sides and lead toward a window or doors at the far end. Curved corridors are an exception to this rule. Because space is often lacking, corridors are also used temporarily to park items such as unused beds, cleaning trolleys or food dispensers, which then stand in corridors and "grace" the entrances to the patient rooms.

Doors

Traditional hospital wards feature monotonous rows of solid, regularly-spaced patient room doors, followed by further similar-looking service room doors. To remedy this, flanking doors for

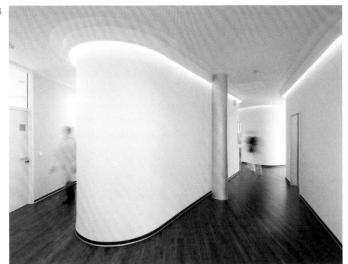

16

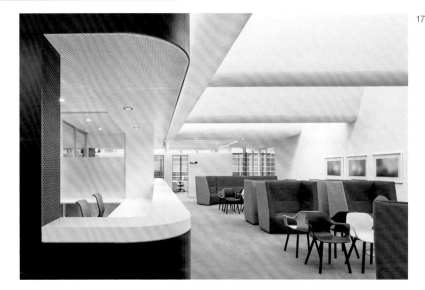

17

14–15   The colours of the walls, windows and ceiling correspond with the colours of the furniture. EwingCole, Children's Hospital of Philadelphia, USA

16   A symbiotic composition of white corridor, curved forms and recessed lighting. Lepel & Lepel, ORTHOPARC Clinic, Cologne, Germany

17   A comfortable waiting area next to a nursing station. Bates Smart, Cabrini Medical Centre, Melbourne, Australia

ancillary functions can be emphasised or alternatively blend into the wall, depending on their purpose, while doors to patient rooms can be articulated as separate entrance areas, for example by grouping them into niches, to reduce the impersonal impression of a mass facility. Respect for patient privacy and their personal space is limited in hospitals; nurses, carers and doctors invariably enter without knocking, partially for time reasons and partially because this is common hospital culture. A good-quality, hotel-like patient room door creates a more positive first impression and denotes the room as personal space, encouraging a more respectful approach to room visits. Tall, double doors heighten this impression by adding a sense of ceremony to entering the room.

Glazed (fire-safety) doors partition wards and corridors, and can be transparent or coated with a one-way foil. Door openers in the form of wall-mounted buttons are placed either side of the doors, sometimes in the form of buzzers to allow staff to control entry and exit. Sensors can also be used to permit or regulate passage and can be advisable in geriatric wards to keep patients in safety, notify staff when patients leave the ward or limit the wandering tendency of dementia sufferers.

Walls

Corridor walls, especially in premium healthcare wards, should present a calm, pleasant backdrop and keep the noise of signs to a minimum. The choice of a coordinated colour scheme and carefully selected works of art or photographs are two suitable approaches. Photographic motifs should avoid showing pictures of wounds, boils, tumours or other illness-related material as they do not help relieve anxiety and promote recovery.

Wall surfaces may simply be white or follow a coordinated colour concept. Painted glass fibre or non-woven wallpaper, or high-quality wall coverings such as patterned or textured wallpapers can also be used to create specific atmospheres. Protective wall coverings on the lower half of walls, and bumper rails and corner guards to protect walls against impact from rolling beds or other trolleys are usually unsightly but in most cases unavoidable. It can be worth trialling a ward without additional protective measures and adding these later only where necessary.

Wall-mounted handrails for patients are a further common feature in corridors and patient wards but are only helpful if they can actually be used, i.e. are not obstructed, which is not always the case. Good-quality wood surfaces are pleasant to touch and hold, and contribute to creating a warm atmosphere.

Floors

As floor coverings typically last a long time, they are usually given a timeless colour. Floor inlays often serve a functional purpose, marking the location of entrances or as wayfinding indicators. Decorative inlays are also used in private healthcare wards. The use of continuous or alternatively contrasting flooring can be used to denote separate areas. In many hospital wards, floors are polished to a shine, as this is held to be synonymous with cleanliness and hygiene. In combination with ceiling lighting, however, this can result in unpleasant reflections. Comfortable patient wards should avoid such typical traits of hospitals. The practice

of polishing floors to achieve the impression of cleanliness is an ongoing problem, especially as incorrect cleaning methods can lead to dirt being "polished" into the floor surface, conserving its presence. Likewise, disinfectant is not always used correctly. This, too, is an ongoing problem. Carpets certified for use in healthcare environments are often used in corridors due to their hotel-like qualities and acoustic damping. However, to clean them, vacuum cleaners are necessary, which introduces a new source of considerable noise.

Ceilings and lighting

Natural illumination, for example from adjoining courtyards, is ideal. Artificial lighting is often incorporated as recessed lighting in easy-to-service suspended ceiling systems that conceal cables and services. Lighting that shines onto side walls creates a more harmonious atmosphere and avoids dazzling patients when transported lying in bed. To reduce costs and save energy, corridor lighting is often switched off, transforming corridors into dim cellar-like tracts. An alternative is energy-efficient LED lighting, which is easy to incorporate and provides a pleasant quality of light that can even adapt to match the time of day.

Lounges

In the context of hospitals, lounges encompass all spaces for patient use outside their room, for example kitchenettes and multifunctional or relaxation spaces. They add variety to the patient's hospital experience, providing an alternative place to receive guests, talk with other patients and enjoy a bite to eat. Tea and fruit are often provided, sometimes also a breakfast buffet. The floors, walls and ceilings should be harmonious in their design, lighting can be decorative and atmospheric, and curtains also help to create an inviting character. Depending on their size, furnishing can be a mix

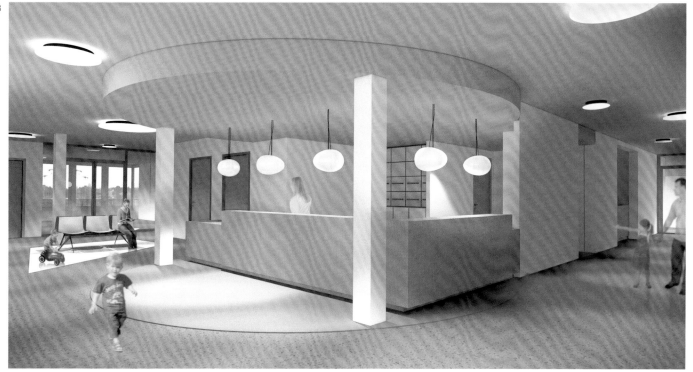

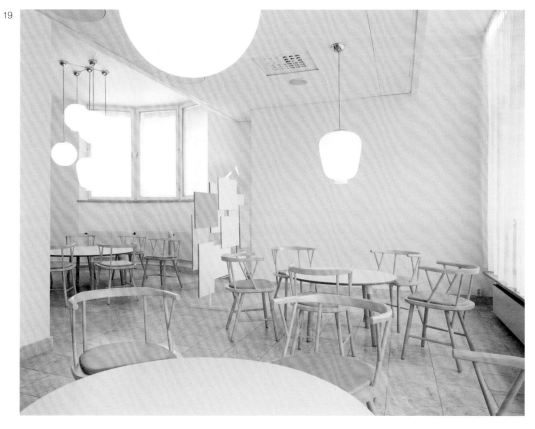

18 The nursing station of this paediatric ward echoes the elements of a child's drawing: green meadows, blue sea and yellow sun. 100% interior Sylvia Leydecker, St. Elisabeth Hospital, Essen, Germany

19 Simple means can also create a friendly impression. TAF, Gabriella Gustafson & Mattias Ståhlbom, Carema Healthcare Center Gullmarsplan, Stockholm, Sweden

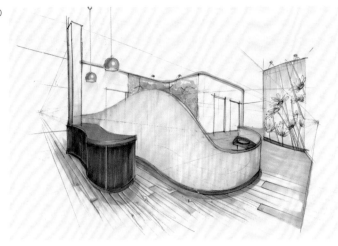

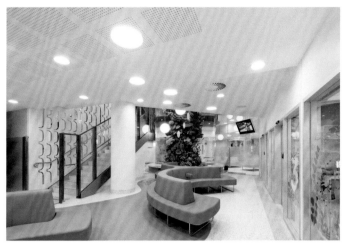

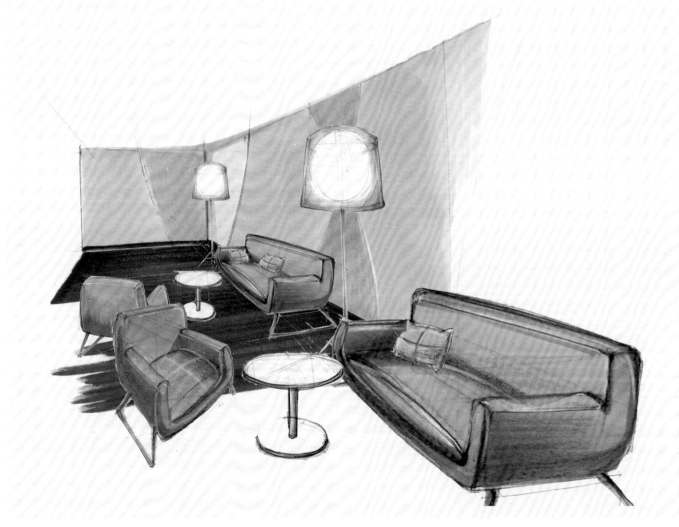

23

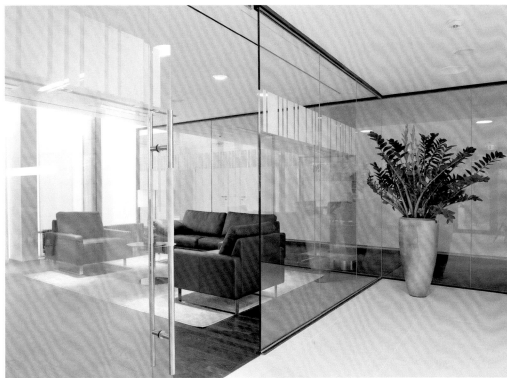

of comfortable sofas and armchairs, reminiscent of a club, and tables and chairs for an additional bistro character.

Which kinds of chairs are most appropriate is a matter for discussion: chairs without armrests are good for mobile patients but less comfortable; armrests, on the other hand, provide support when getting up. Square or rectangular tables have the advantage that several can be combined to form a larger table. Round tables lack this benefit, but look better in haphazard arrangements, unlike square tables which look untidy when not lined up. High tables can be good for patients for whom sitting is uncomfortable; walking aid holders are also advisable. In sum, lounges should provide comfortable, home-like areas that have a private feel to them and an inviting sense of comfort and quality.

Waiting areas

Waiting areas can have quite different characters. There is a huge difference between a waiting room in accidents and emergencies with a high through-put of patients and the comparatively relaxed waiting area to see the head doctor. For the lat-ter, a couple of comfortable armchairs, a coffee machine, perhaps with background music, eases the typically short wait. The rows of chairs in the corridors of the accidents and emergencies depart-ment, by contrast, are more reminiscent of an air-port lounge, arranged for optimum fire safety. Even so, they can still be comfortable and a welcoming sight. Loose items of furniture tend to meander about the room as patients move chairs and tables. As hospitals have no equivalent to a hotel house-keeper to ensure everything is put back in place,

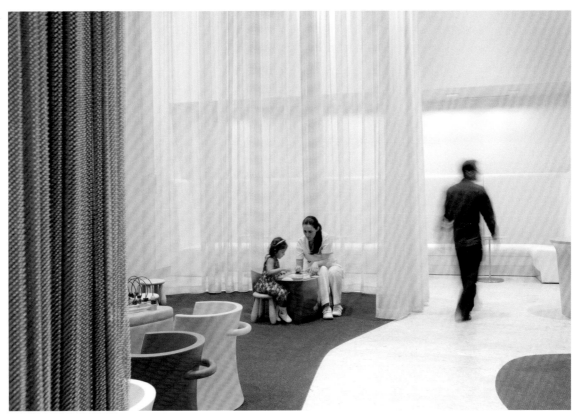

this can at times result in a rather disorderly impression. Cost is also a factor as more comfortable chairs are generally more expensive. Visitors appreciate seating with some degree of upholstering, for example armchairs of the kind found on cruise ships or in better restaurants. Given the rising levels of obesity, it can be advisable to also provide suitably robust seats, discreetly disguised as twin seats.

A thoughtful design concept for waiting rooms can lend these transitory spaces a character and definition of their own. Extending this principle to other wards with slight variations can turn a "boring" activity into a varied experience and help give identity to the different parts of the hospital. TV screens serve as a welcome diversion that subjectively shortens the waiting time and reduces the amount of questions that staff have to field. Changes in floor surfacing can be used to subtly mark off specific areas according to activity, to reduce the hustle and bustle of visitors coming and going. Other circulation spaces – entrances, lift lobbies, etc. – generally precede waiting areas and likewise need appropriate design consideration, for example through the placement of seating and the design of the wall surfaces and lighting. A designated space or holders for brochures and reading material should be provided to prevent paper spreading around the room.

Reception areas and nursing stations

Arriving patients should ideally be greeted by schooled staff in a reception area with an open and approachable character that avoids creating barriers between visitors and staff. The services that take place at the reception set the tone for the rest

24 A stylish waiting area for young
   patients and their parents. NBBJ,
   Dubai Mall Medical Centre, United
   Arab Emirates

25–26 Geometric arrangements of
   coloured surfaces extend across
   the walls and ceiling of these waiting
   areas. raumkontor Innenarchitektur,
   Manus Clinic, Krefeld, Germany

27 The wall appears to recede and dis-
   solve to reveal the reception area.
   TAF, Gabriella Gustafson & Mattias
   Ståhlbom, Carema Healthcare
   Center Gullmarsplan, Stockholm,
   Sweden

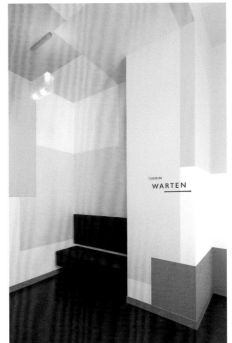
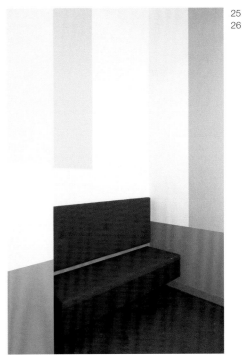

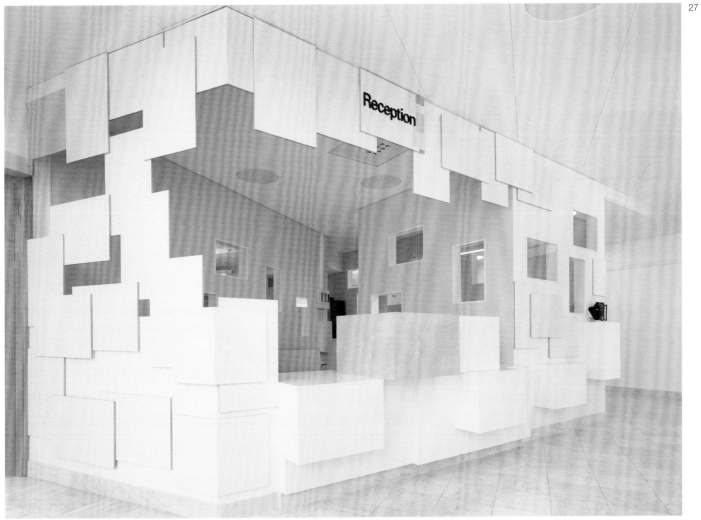

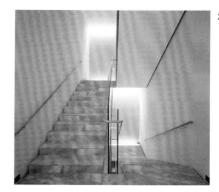

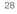

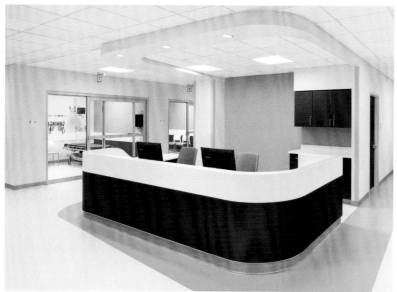

of the hospital visit for patients and visitors alike. While an attractive and inviting design creates a conducive environment, it cannot replace friendly and attentive staff. The necessary admission procedures should ideally take place in a separate room for greater discretion and to ensure data protection, the latter being especially important in healthcare institutions.

These principles apply equally to the design of nursing stations, which, for fire safety reasons, are all too often more akin to railway station ticket counters hidden behind safety glass. Nursing stations are not only a patient's first port of call on arrival in a ward. They are also the point from which the patient is discharged: here too they should leave with a positive impression.

Summary: The consideration of all these diverse aspects, always with the patient's recovery in mind, helps lead to comfortable environments that complement and support top-quality medical care. The interior architecture of healing environments can benefit all its users: good hospital interiors promote an atmosphere of well-being, which in turn has a reciprocal effect on staff behaviour and patient satisfaction.

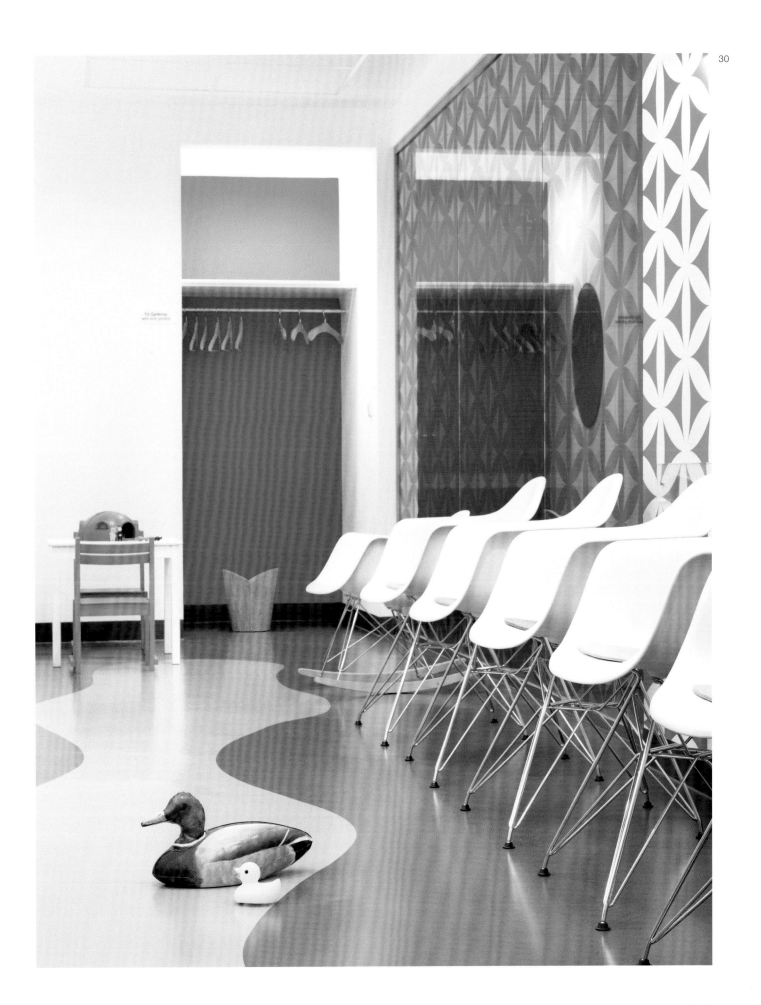

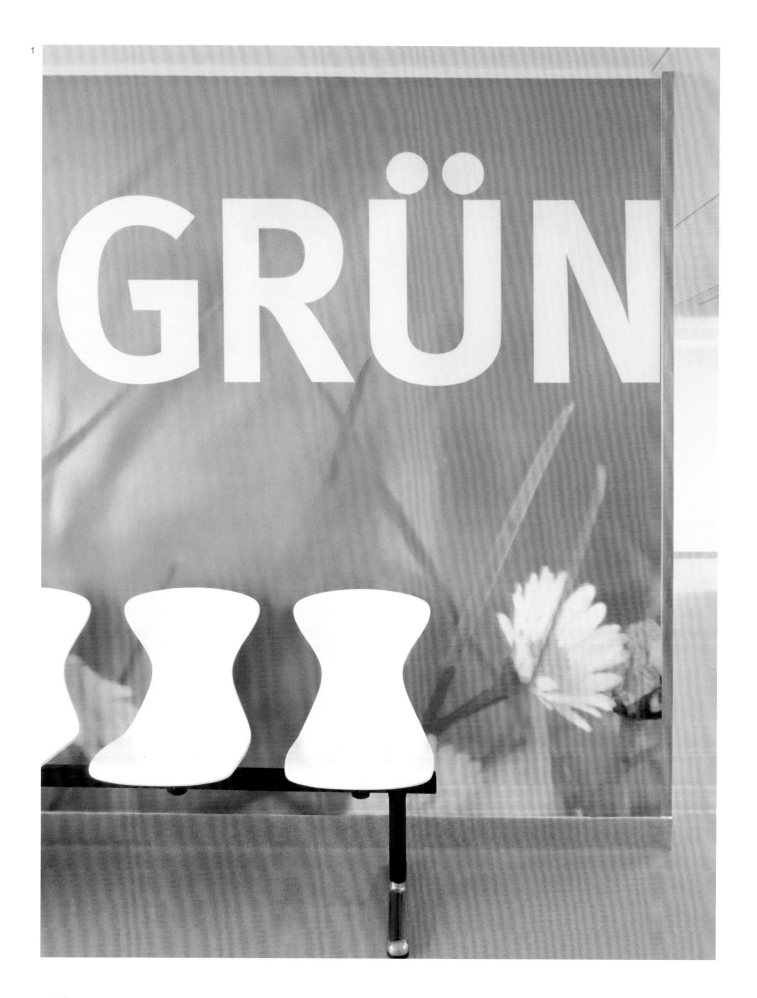

1

Key components of the design task

1 Inspirational design elements can turn a simple waiting area in a large clinic into a moment of peace and tranquillity for anxious patients. 100% interior Sylvia Leydecker, Heidelberg University Hospital, Germany

A complex design task

Designing a patient room is considerably more complex than it at first seems. While the arrangement of a bed, bedside table, lamp, cupboard, table and chair may appear relatively straightforward, the task of designing a patient room befitting of its purpose is more complex and goes far beyond these basic components. Numerous aspects need to be considered including the optimisation of processes, efficient use of space, sensible working systems, hygiene requirements and ease of cleaning, and cost effectiveness with respect to both the initial investment and later maintenance. These functional and economic concerns are all fundamental aspects. In addition, patient rooms should ideally also respond to emotional needs, support patient well-being, fulfil aesthetic expectations and be marketable for the various stakeholders involved.

How is this achieved in practice? Aside from the arrangement of the floor plan, which must consider use patterns and facilitate the smooth execution of typical tasks, the key design components of a patient room and associated areas are primarily material, colour, form and light. The design must always consider the overall effect and wider context. No single component can be considered in isolation because it is always part of its built context. Changing one component has a corresponding effect on the whole, and changing the context changes the overall effect.

Design quality

Good-quality design responds to the required functionality with clearly arranged floor plans, sensible progressions of spaces and clearly organised pathways. A construction method appropriate to the material, including all relevant details, facili-

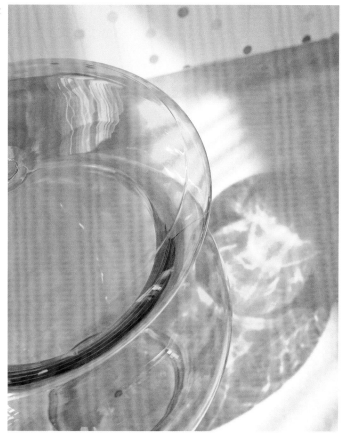

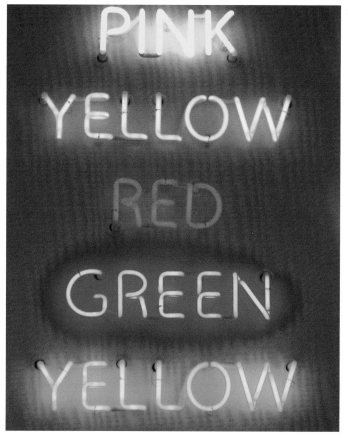

tates efficient on-site construction and ensures that the end result properly reflects the plans. Likewise, the qualities of materials and products should not only look good and fulfil their purpose, but also be durable and age well without becoming unsightly. The material concept should harmonise with the colour concept and be augmented by the lighting concept. Details such as the sensible positioning of light switches and handles, the articulation of clean lines and the consideration of views inside and out as well as pathways through spaces help give spaces a sense of calm clarity.

An example of the opposite is the maze of signs that adorn some hospital walls in myriad formats, colours, typefaces, some home-made, some painted, tacked on with strips of sticky plaster in a haphazard arrangement. Considering the overall design in this context means incorporating these different signage needs into an organised system of wayfinding with signage elements that complement rather than dictate the design concept of the architecture and interior architecture. Wayfinding

systems often employ colours as a means of denoting location. But while these may be functional and attractive, they also have to be appropriate to the desired atmosphere of the respective areas. For example, the bold colours often used to aid orientation in car parks do not always harmonise with the psychological needs of patients.

Colour

Colours that we perceive as being pleasant have a positive effect on the atmosphere of our environments. The colour concept influences the mood of spaces – pleasantly calming or subtly stimulating, uplifting for the spirit or supportive of bodily functions – and can serve as an aid and positive force. But if used without care, it can feel uncoordinated, bewildering, disorientating or busy; it can cause emotional distress or even anxiety or depression. The colour concept is therefore one of the most vital components of the interior design.

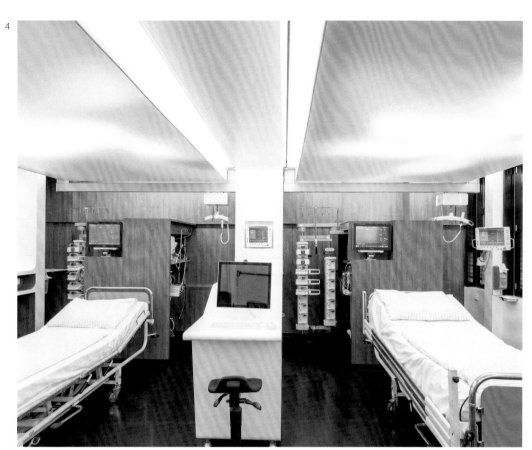

4

2   Sunlight reflecting off a simple transparent acrylic stool enlivens a space. 100% interior Sylvia Leydecker, Rems-Murr Hospital, Winnenden, Germany

3   Colour and light are key design components.

4   Research project for a patient-centred intensive care room with illuminated ceiling panels, reduced noise levels and concealed equipment. GRAFT Architekten, (T)Raumgestaltung, Campus Virchow-Clinic, Charité, Berlin, Germany

Most discussions on attractive interiors in healthcare environments revolve around the colour concept, to the neglect of other contributing design aspects. It is a subject that everyone has an opinion on, and advice abounds: bright, warm, friendly, invigorating, inviting, and restful are just some of the typical attributes that a good room design should have, so one is told. Not surprisingly, colour concepts that correspond to these attributes – yellow and apricot with a hint of terracotta or dark red as accent colours – are popular among hospital operators. Hospital colour concepts also go through trends: white and surgical green gave way to petrol and pastel yellow, then to "feel-good" colours such as apricot, yellow and terracotta, then to trendy colours such as apple green, which remains a firm favourite among marketing departments.

White is almost always perceived as being too "sterile" and has predominantly negative connotations. This need not necessarily be the case: white has its place and can even express the opposite of sterile, depending on the context. For example,

naturally-lit spaces with wooden floors and white, not too smooth walls result in pleasant, bright and light interiors that are calm and unfussy, and contrast pleasingly with the world outside – ideal environments for both recovering while looking out over nature and for concentrated work. This contrast is more effective with a lighter white than a pale yellow or apricot.

Signal colours such as petrol or orange are firm favourites for hospital logos as well as interiors. The effect can be dramatic, especially when used for a before-and-after makeover (i.e. a cost-effective repaint) of a ward. Bold and varied colours are, however, often more difficult to maintain in the long term than a more discreet colour concept. As a rule, stronger, striking colours are better used as accents, for example a single dark red wall surface. Likewise, it is better to avoid using such colours on very durable surfaces such as floor coverings that will remain in place for a long time. Here the choice of a neutral, timeless colour affords greater flexibility in future.

The perception of colours changes with the ambient lighting conditions: natural light has an optimum colour spectrum, whereas artificial light varies, often exhibiting a shift towards reds or blues in the colour spectrum. How colours are perceived also varies with the surface quality, for example if textured or shiny. Colours also affect how other objects are perceived: a light-coloured armchair appears lighter in weight against a sky-blue background than a night-blue background. Colours are associated with smells, as in the case of violet or yellow, for instance, and some colours have gender-specific associations: black, for example, is broad and vigorous, and therefore perceived as typically masculine, whereas pink is considered delicate and feminine. Care should be taken with reflective colour surfaces, for example a green or red wall, as these can alter how we see – and diagnose – skin tones. Materials can also change how we perceive colours: wood, glass, plastic, etc. can all create colour shifts, and some colours also change over time with aging. All these aspects need to be taken into consideration.

To achieve a harmonious overall impression, colours therefore need to be carefully coordinated and specified. The names of colours are unreliable as indicators of their actual colour: white can range from snow white to cream, and grey varies from light grey to warm anthracite. Similar colours can clash and it is important to compare paints from different manufacturers. Do colours conform to standard colour specifications, or are they from the supplier's own range? Will they still be available in future? And will there be small variations in colour between manufacturing batches, for example when ordering smaller quantities for replacement floor covering at a later date? Such questions are also relevant for the colour concept, as even slight colour differences become apparent when used in combination.

Material authenticity

There is no material without colour, whether immanent to the material or artificial. The debate on material authenticity in hospital design often revolves around the question of whether to use natural wood or wood-effect materials. Some categorically reject the artificiality of the imitation while others not only merely accept but actively embrace its qualities. The artificial material addresses the wish for a classier, hotel-like, warmer and homely atmosphere while fulfilling hygiene requirements and being easy to clean. Natural wood indisputably adds a special atmosphere that sets it apart from typical sterile hospital interiors, but as an organic material it does not fulfil hygiene requirements without at least one layer of varnish. That explains the popularity of imitation wood surfaces. Authentic materials such as natural wood (although in end effect more often a veneer) cannot offer the same range of properties. Natural wood floors require elaborate, extensive varnishing, but here too a scratch is the equivalent of a crater for bacteria. Furniture veneer is likewise relatively sensitive. This, along with the lower cost, is the reason why imitation wood surface materials are routinely used in the design of patient rooms.

In the design of furniture, the edge detail is an interesting case: a simple glue-on cover strip, a more durable Acryl-Butadien-Styrol (ABS) edging strip or a seamless edge design all communicate different impressions of authenticity. Other details such as the thickness of shelf boards or the kind and quality of fittings, hinges, runners and knobs can differ significantly with respect to material, hygiene and load capacity. Here too, materials are not always as authentic as they look. Chrome surfaces or brushed aluminium may turn out to be coated plastic, whereby the quality of the plastic determines how convincing the impression is. The same phenomenon can be seen even in high-class automobile interiors: in many cases the supposedly metal or carbon fibre trim is an imitation of such good quality that the owner rarely notices. Imitation leather upholstery that looks like real leather is used widely both in hospital furnishings and for car upholstery.

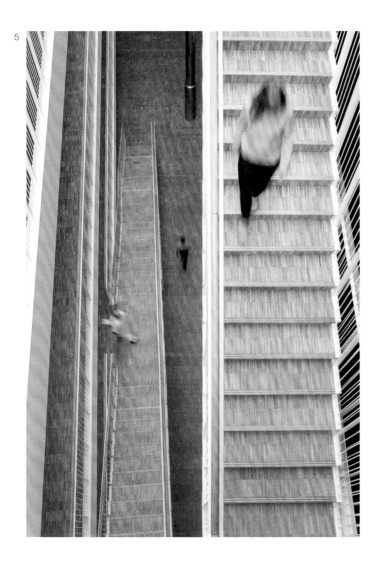

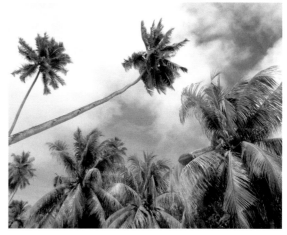

7

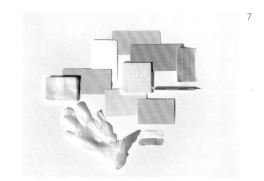

8

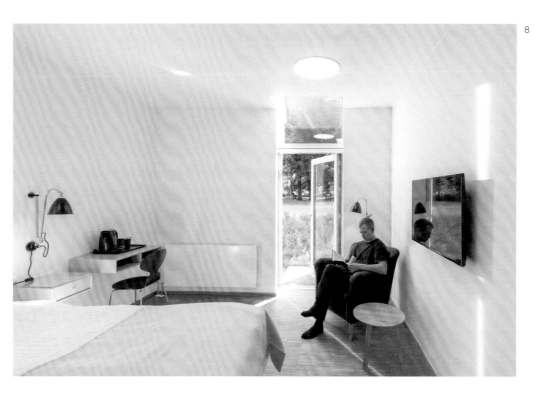

5 Real wood flooring and open, airy interiors lend spaces a natural quality. 3XN, Rigshospitalet, Copenhagen, Denmark

6 Whether German pine forests or Caribbean palm trees, a view of greenery does patients good.

7 A material collage with sunny accents. TAF, Gabriella Gustafson & Mattias Ståhlbom, Carema Healthcare Center Gullmarsplan, Stockholm, Sweden

8 Clean lines, contrasting black and white surfaces, wood and grass. Rigshospitalet

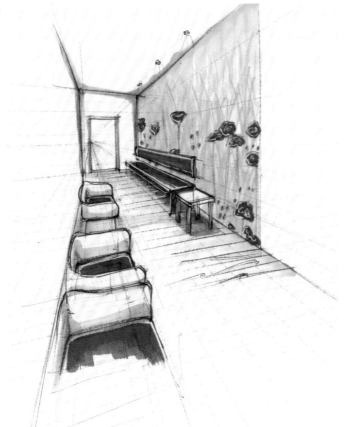

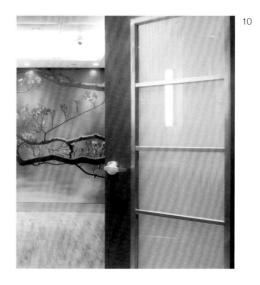

In the interior fittings, floor coverings and the laminated faces of furniture are the primary surfaces. They not only imitate wood surfaces but also textiles, metal and concrete, complete with patina if required, although rust and weathered wood is less appropriate for hospital contexts. The range of imitation materials is remarkably diverse, spanning from artificial fibres that imitate wool or silk to stained maple with an exotic dark colour and transparent plastics that look at first glance like glass. Major technological advances in the industrial production of artificial materials and the resulting products have made them ever more difficult to differentiate from the original. The decision for or against a particular product or material is frequently a question of weighing up functional requirements such as durability, ease of cleaning, hygiene (easy to wipe down, resistant to disinfectants, impervious to urine) and fire safety against comfort, aesthetics, emotional response and cost-effectiveness.

The cost factor begins in some cases with the production costs, whereby this is a matter for the industry. The newest innovations from the manufacturers' R&D labs are of little use if they are too expensive. Ultimately, companies need sales to survive. For the design of premium patient rooms in healthcare wards, this will mean that it should not be necessary to choose between good-quality door fittings or good-quality bedding – both should ideally be possible.

Multi-sensory design

Multi-sensory perception – i.e. how we perceive environments with all our senses – is extremely complex and takes place subconsciously within a fraction of a second. To date it has not yet been fully researched. What we do know is that the brain receives and processes millions of impulses almost instantaneously, but the precise mechanisms of how this functions are the subject of ongoing brain research. For the design of patient rooms, this means that designers and architects should consider all the senses and how they can be influenced, and not just the visual appearance

The means available to influence people's behaviour through multi-sensory design are extensive, and in extreme cases can be deliberately and blatantly manipulative. Neuropsychology is already used successfully in other product marketing sectors to increase sales. In practice, the idea is not as complicated as it may sound: addressing particular senses triggers "brainscripts" which people in turn associate with specific experiences. For example, Italian music is a better match when buying spaghetti than heavy metal; a hint of perfume in the bedroom is more arousing than the smell of sausages. Similarly, the sound of waves lapping gently evokes pleasant sensations of the sea, the smell of freshly-baked cookies signals the cosiness of Christmastime and birdsong a spring morning. These mechanisms can likewise be used in hospitals to trigger positive associations: hence the frequent use of images of woods, meadows and flowers. Rooms can evoke associations with other worlds and tell stories. Here design is not

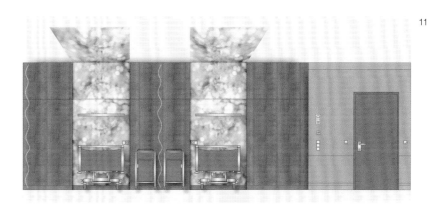

11

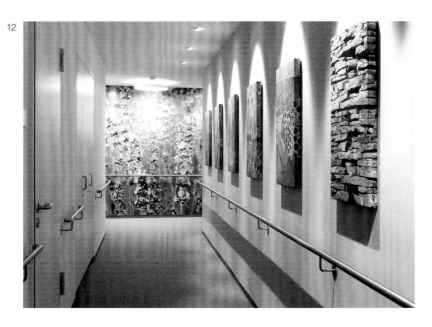

12

9   Images of red poppies on the wall enliven a waiting area. 100% interior Sylvia Leydecker, Radiological Health-care Centre Minden-Löhne, Germany

10   Cherry blossoms welcome one into the entrance area. e4h architecture, Lenox Hill Hospital, New York, USA

11   Bright green foliage as a backdrop for the patients is calming and relaxing. 100% interior Sylvia Leydecker, St. Vinzenz Hospital, Düsseldorf, Germany

12   Creative interpretations of lavender establish a visual and mental connection between the internal corridor and the garden outside. 100% interior Sylvia Leydecker, Hospice of the Foundation Marien Hospital, Euskirchen, Germany

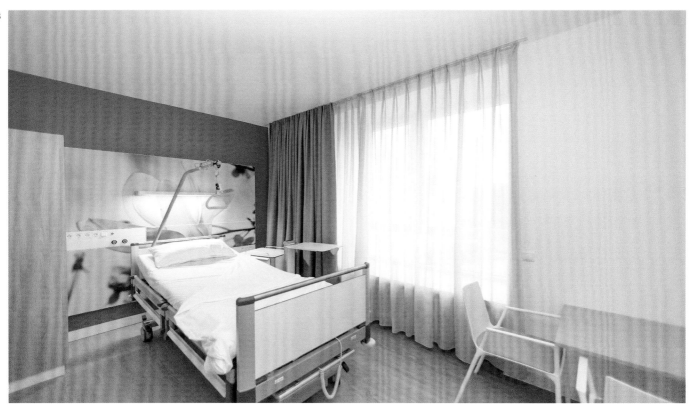

about manipulation but considering how patient and visitor well-being can be improved by designing for all the senses. The most relevant senses in this context are the visual, acoustic, haptic, tactile and olfactory senses.

Haptic

Haptic qualities make a comparatively subtle contribution to the atmosphere of a space. How something feels, whether registered consciously or subconsciously, can be a pleasing experience. It can be soft and gentle, firm to hold or slippery, rough and unpleasant, or smooth and mysterious like a stone made of Netsuke plastic. Finely differentiated surfaces are used in psychosomatic therapy to

consciously focus attention on the senses. Sensing different structures and textures can be an exercise in mindfulness. Surfaces one holds or touches are therefore typical candidates for haptic treatment. In geriatric wards, for example, different surface textures can be used to mark locations along a handrail, such as the entry to rooms.

The haptic qualities of the floor are felt underfoot rather than by touch: ceramic tiles or stone paving are hard, carpets (certified for healthcare use) are soft, while wood is warm. Fall prevention is an important aspect for all areas, not just geriatric wards, primarily to prevent injury, but also to reduce hospital liability claims and the costs and reputational damage this can cause. Floor surfaces must therefore be designed with appropriate anti-slip qualities to prevent people from stumbling or slipping. As rough, anti-slip surfaces compromise the hygienic continuity of smooth surfaces, the designer must weigh up the respective needs according to priority in the different areas.

Switches, handles and grips are constantly being touched and can therefore have haptic qualities. While this is commonly taken into consideration in the design of door handles and grips, it is invariably neglected in the design of light switches. Touch simultaneously involves sensing surface temperature: plastic is warmer to the touch than steel or glass, which can be unpleasantly cool. For this reason, wooden handrails are always preferred over steel, as are aluminium door fittings, as both materials are warmer and more pleasant to touch than steel.

Indoor air quality – temperature

Room temperature can be an ongoing point of contention in two-bed rooms as people have sometimes significantly different temperature sensitivities and fresh air needs. Is the room temperature pleasant? Does it get too hot when the sun shines? Or arctically cold when the air conditioning is on? Sun shades and smart materials such as latent heat accumulators/PCMs (Phase Change Materials) can be used to buffer high and low temperature extremes, keeping the room at a pleasant temperature. These materials can be incorporated in wall constructions, for example in the form of micro-capsules embedded in plaster or plasterboard with a wax filling that changes from solid to liquid, and vice versa, within a defined temperature

14

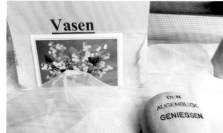

15

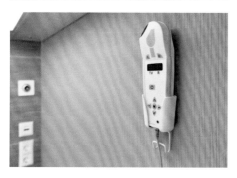

16

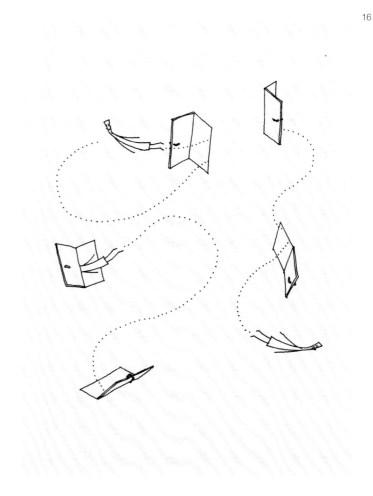

13 Images of nature evoke positive associations. Bernd Kirchbrücher, raumlinq Gmbh, Caritas Hospital, Bad Mergentheim, Germany

14 Well-meaning still life in a hospital

15 Easy-to-use remote controls

within easy reach of the patient are an indispensable feature in the design of premium patient rooms. 100% interior Sylvia Leydecker, Rems-Murr Hospital, Winnenden, Germany

16 Sketch of the patient in the hospital process. nendo, MD.net Clinic, Tokyo, Japan

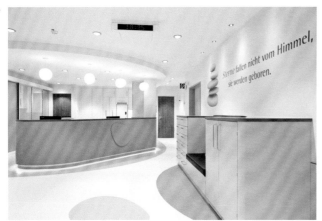

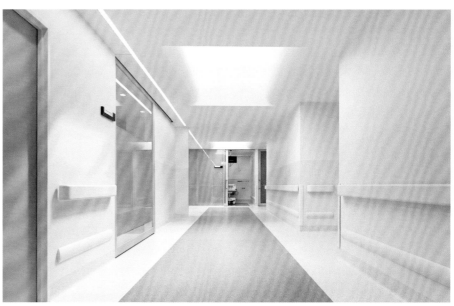

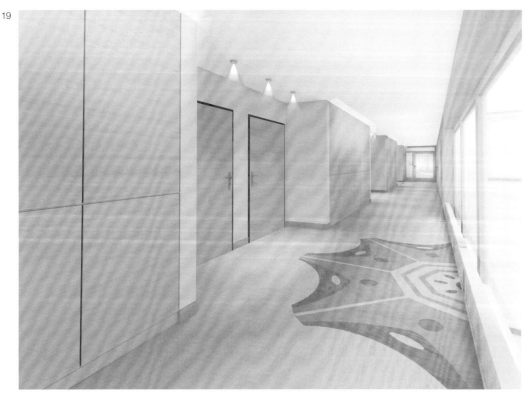

17 Reception area with stress-free wellness character in a maternity ward. 100% interior Sylvia Leydecker, Elisabeth Hospital, Essen, Germany

18 A clean and pleasant corridor space. Bates Smart, Cabrini Medical Centre, Melbourne, Australia

19 An elaborate floor inlay as a special feature in a circulation space. 100% interior Sylvia Leydecker, Rems-Murr Hospital, Schorndorf, Germany

range. This so-called phase change either absorbs or gives off energy, thereby buffering changes in the room temperature.

Indoor air quality – smell

Smells in hospitals are often a combination of the usually unpleasant smell of disinfectant and warm food. Good air quality is not necessarily just the absence of unpleasant odours but also the presence of pleasant smells. In most patient rooms, fresh air is desirable and indicates that the room is looked after. Flowers can also help speed recovery. Fragrant blossoms and blends of incense have been used for thousands of years to raise spirits. However, artificial room fragrances should be used with care as they are often unnecessary and can cause allergic reactions among some patients.

Smells can also arise through the introduction of new materials. Various materials emit volatile substances, which generally dissipate after a short while. Refurbishment work on existing wards can make this more apparent.

Smells as indicators of pollutants

In some cases, smells alert to the fact that materials contain substances, for example formaldehyde, that emit unhealthy or potentially toxic substances into the room air. They diffuse from products and materials and can sometimes cause intense reactions. Staff who are permanently exposed to such emissions are particularly at risk. Some instances of Sick Building Syndrome (SBS) have even led to buildings being declared unfit for use.

Floor coverings

Hospitals have potentially millions of square metres of flooring, making it vital to carefully assess the available options. Linoleum is regarded as a very natural floor covering, as is natural rubber, provided it has a European EPD (Environmental Product Declaration). Vinyl flooring is available in phthalate-free varieties mixed with natural materials such as cork to reduce the PVC content. Petrochemical-based raw materials should gradually be replaced in favour of products made from renewable raw materials, and coatings are continually being optimised. The absence of chlorine is important for fire safety reasons. The surface areas involved in hospitals can be vast.

Aside from the floor covering itself, the adhesive used to apply it is also relevant, as are the quantities of adhesive required – some non-hazardous materials can nevertheless exceed statutory limits when used in very large quantities. Likewise, care should be taken to avoid material combinations that can react chemically with each other. Flooring system providers know which different system components – floor covering, adhesive and coating – are compatible and function well together, and specify them accordingly. This has gained increasing importance in the context of concerns regarding the indoor air quality of hospitals.

Ultimately, a patient room is not a laboratory, and interior architects and designers are not experts in chemistry. For the physical well-being of patients, the indoor air quality of patient rooms can be improved through ventilation, air conditioning, the choice of materials and cleaning.

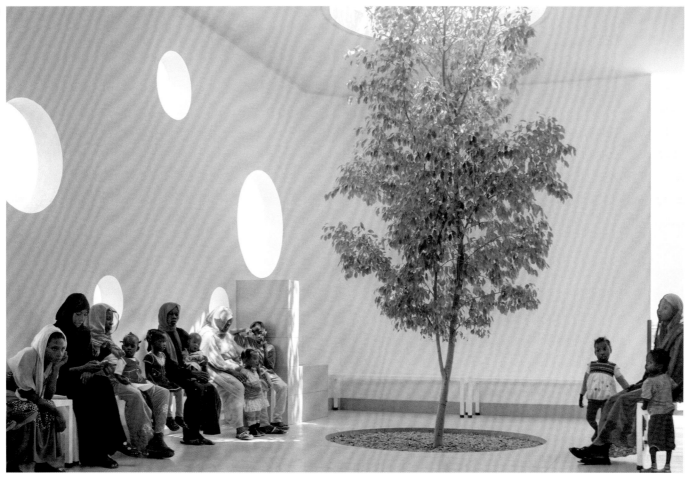

Sustainability and the environment

Sustainability makes itself most evident in usability and in usage. Sustainability is not always about maximising efficiency; it is also about sufficiency. Much of what we need can be achieved with less input and fewer resources – isn't this in many ways the most promising approach for the future? Accordingly, current hospital design places increasing importance on incorporating greater flexibility for better long-term sustainability.

Rooms should be able to adapt to changing processes. If a key parameter changes, it can alter the requirements, making it necessary to find a new solution. While it is not possible to predict all future parameters, not least because a single parameter can cause a fundamental shift in the system, it is possible, with the help of prognoses and flexible solutions, to be as well-equipped as possible for changing circumstances. To paraphrase Darwin, not the strongest but the most adaptable survive. Design therefore needs to embrace the principles of responsiveness and flexibility.

In response to increasing environmental pollution and rising costs as a consequence of depleting resources, designers are being called on to be more ecologically conscious. Ecological materials and products suitable for use in hospital interiors are now increasingly being manufactured at scale and therefore becoming affordable. Products made of renewable raw materials that require fewer finite resources for their production, that are energy-efficient and produced under fair conditions by companies from the region that take corporate social responsibility seriously and abhor greenwashing are desirable. Innovative products, whether furniture, materials for furniture, coatings, upholstery, floor coverings, wallpapers, paints, curtains or lights, are gradually making significant inroads into the market. The industry is constantly developing new technologies, improving production methods, optimising their products and adding new possibilities.

In most cases, products and materials are typically considered only in their end state. Little thought is given to the entire lifecycle, to the previous life (the energy-intensive production process) and the later life (the demolition, disposal and recycling) of products, although these are just as important. Certificates and labels such as the well-established "Blue Angel" or the "EPD Environmental Product Declarations", or the newer DGNB (Deutsche Gesellschaft für Nachhaltiges Bauen e.V.) label are reliable indicators and provide orientation for designers and specifiers. Demand is increasing for products that conserve resources, that have a small carbon footprint in the overall energy balance, and likewise for cradle-to-cradle (as opposed to cradle-to-grave) approaches. In all cases, the raw material should generally be non-hazardous.

The building industry is slow to take up new innovations, not least due to building product approval, the relevant norms and liability risks. Innovative products take a while to make it onto the market and are therefore more expensive than comparable standard products. More often than not, they lose out in tendering to more economical products, and are therefore only rarely put into practice.

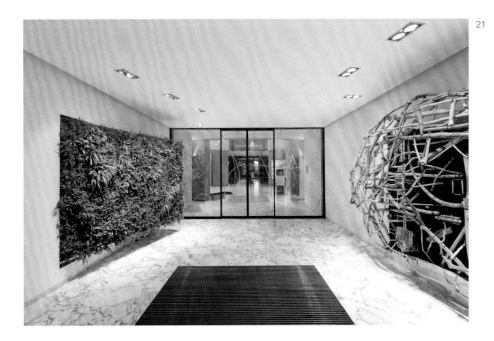

21

20   Simple, circular openings and a tree establish a connection between inside and outside. TAMassociati, Paediatric Centre, Port Sudan, Sudan

21   A green "living wall" positioned opposite an art installation lends drama to this entrance space. Schmucker und Partner, Ethianum Clinic, Heidelberg, Germany.

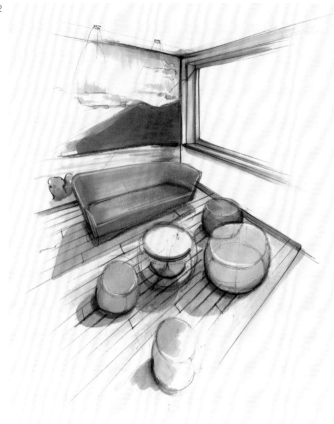

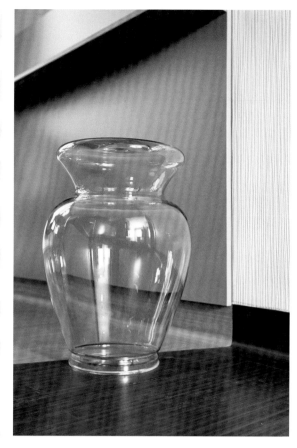

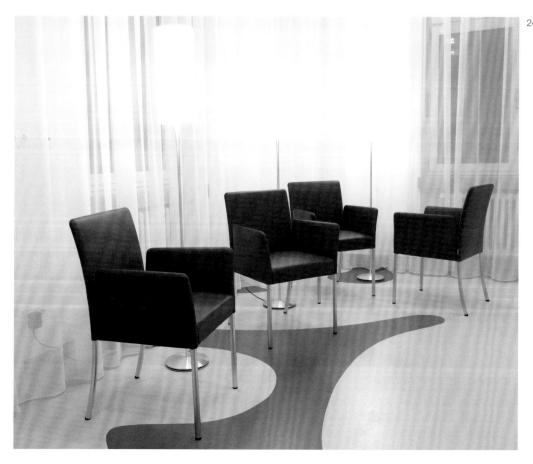

22 "Out of the blue" – sketch of a relaxing lounge with a corresponding acoustic atmosphere. 100% interior Sylvia Leydecker, Radiological Healthcare Centre Minden-Löhne, Germany

23 A plastic stool and clean junction details make it easier to maintain good hygiene. 100% interior Sylvia Leydecker, Rems-Murr Hospital, Winnenden, Germany

24 Seamless floor inlays add atmospheric touches while remaining hygienic. 100% interior Sylvia Leydecker, Private Clinic Josephinum, Munich, Germany

Good-quality products have their price but are often sidelined in favour of comparable (clone) products or even plagiarisms that cost less. This reveals a problem with neutral tendering procedures that limit the incidence of objections and the associated delays these cause. Objections are used to contest the awarding of a contract to a competitor, often by exploiting inconsistencies or gaps in the tendering documents. Regardless of the quality of the product or its innovative potential, environmental concerns rarely have a higher priority than the investment cost.

Construction details

Where surfaces that enclose a space meet, detailing is critical. A case in point is the junction between the base of a wall and the floor: a cove profile in which the floor surface curves seamlessly upwards and extends up the wall is ideal for easy cleaning and hygiene, but must be well-executed to avoid material cracking, especially at the corners of rooms. However, this is not always practical: a vinyl floor covering with a wood-effect finish will look wrong turning up the wall.

Seams and cracks represent huge points of attack for germs and bacteria, and careful detailing is required to prevent them occurring. Junctions between sections of flooring are also critical as uncontrollable gaps can arise, in which dirt collects and mould can form. Natural wood floors, even when varnished, can get scratched, creating the equivalent of valleys for germs. Silicone joints require regular maintenance in locations where mould and bacteria have ideal, warm and moist conditions. Ideally all cracks, gaps and crevices should be avoided, likewise all hard-to-reach areas where dirt can collect such as on top of cupboards or fittings that don't quite reach the ceiling, in the joints in furniture that is not screwed together properly or in gaps between sections of upholstery.

Sound

The acoustic impression of a space – its sound so to speak – affects its atmosphere more than one might think and therefore requires due consideration.

Lots of sounds are heard in patient rooms: conversations, the TV, coughing, footfalls in the corridor, items clattering, the sound of cleaning, voices and so on. Medical equipment also produces noises. The predominance of hard, sound-reflecting surfaces such as the smooth surfaces of furniture and the floor in combination with large-format glazing can create unpleasant acoustic reverberations. Reverberations affect the clarity with which one can hear things. The sound of a floor covering when walked on heightens this effect and can contribute to the atmosphere of a space, for example soft steps on carpets or loud steps on ceramic tiles, depending on the type of shoe sole.

Often different needs and requirements conflict: for example, large windows that look onto gardens are desirable and constitute a key part of a healing environment. At the same time, however, they contribute to the reverberant atmosphere of the room, requiring other compensatory measures to optimise the acoustics.

Acoustics

Noise and commotion are not conducive to relaxation and recovery and hence disrupt the patient's process of regaining health. For staff, ongoing noise is stressful too, and can make people ill in the long term. While peace and quiet is pleasant, absolute silence is not. Patients require a level of sound around them, ideally of human origin, to feel looked after and not alone and forlorn. Acoustic materials can be used to counteract the effects of excess noise. Acoustic ceilings in foyers, for example, or acoustic plasters and panels on walls can effectively reduce the transmission of airborne sound. Sound-insulated doors can reduce sound intrusion and contribute to a sense of privacy.

Privacy screening

The need for privacy in private healthcare patient rooms begins with permission to enter a private area. In normal cases, patient rooms can be entered immediately. Special areas such as a private lounge area or comfort wards may require possession of an RFID (radio-frequency identification) tag to allow entry. In extreme cases, some patients are protected by bodyguards and only move around within the bounds of a defined space. Frosted glass prevents people outside from looking in. A similar situation arises where separate blocks or wings of a hospital overlook one another. Here curtains or blinds are commonly used to ensure privacy. Within the actual patient room, curtains can afford privacy in two-bed rooms or when treatments or use of a bedpan are necessary while relatives are in the room. At the most basic level, therefore, a simple screen can ensure discretion and provide a modicum of privacy.

Light

Interior architects must consider both artificial light and natural light. Artificial lighting can be functional, i.e. assist orientation, provide light for examinations and diagnoses, or atmospheric light for a sense of well-being.

Natural light is essential for patient well-being. It structures the course of the day from morning until night as the red and the blue component of the light varies and influences people's biorhythm. So-called circadian lighting is sometimes used in hospitals to artificially simulate the natural rhythm of the day. Strong daylight may require blinds or shading systems to filter glare and bright light to a softer level. Ideally, patients should be able to comfortably control the incidence of natural light from their bed.

Artificial light is essential for examinations and diagnosis, where it must provide a defined nominal

25

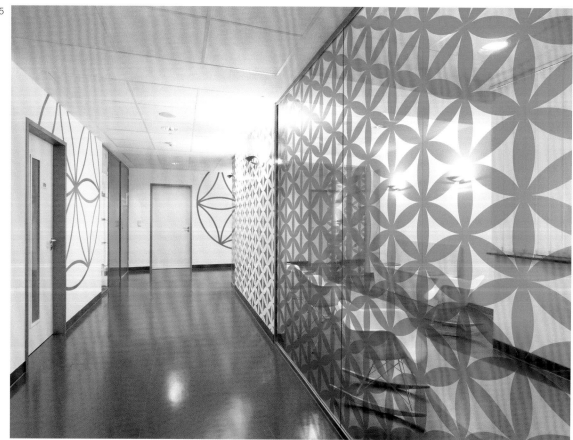

illuminance. Atmospheric lighting, by contrast, requires different kinds of lighting and lighting scenarios, using a combination of accent lighting, spot lights, wall washers that light up and highlight surfaces, and so on. These must be hygienic and easy to clean without using too many different light sources that over-complicate facility management. LEDs are now widely used as an efficient form of lighting. A separately adjustable reading lamp for patients is practical. To reduce the risk of falls, low-level night-lights are advisable, and if not permanently on, can be triggered by a motion sensor. LEDs have become the standard preferred light source due to their low energy consumption. The use of a limited number of different light sources is recommended for easier maintenance.

Smart applications

Developments in lighting technology are increasingly overlapping with advances in IT. Illuminated OLED foils and panels with interactive touch-sensitive surfaces are one example of such crossover products. Microsystems with sensors and digital controllers for various functions herald the arrival of the smart patient room. These controllers will make it possible for patients to adjust room temperature, open and close doors, raise and lower blinds, change room lighting and also to operate the entertainment centre – whether on the wall or at the bedside – with TV, VOD (Video on Demand), music, games and Internet.

Digital patient records combined with virtual remote diagnosis are a further upcoming development. The ability to easily control the entire range of relevant functions makes it possible to interlink different systems, but requires suitable interfaces between

26

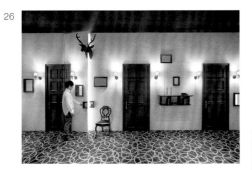

27

25 A translucent partition with graphic ornaments acts as a screen while reducing the sense of enclosure in the waiting area. 100% interior Sylvia Leydecker, Obstetrics Unit, Maria-Hilf Hospital, Brilon, Germany

26–27 An unusual perspective in a psychiatric clinic. Opening the door opens an entire section of the wall. nendo, MD.net Clinic, Tokyo, Japan

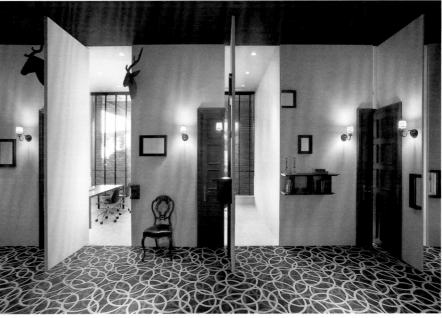

28 Different kinds of indirect lighting
are essential for creating atmospheric interiors. dwp, Jaypee
Medical Centre, Noida, India

29 Ample daylight creates an
attractive place to be. The colour
of the interior fittings corresponds with the glazed sections of
the façade. 100% interior
Sylvia Leydecker, Rems-Murr
Hospital, Winnenden, Germany

30 Smart controls make it possible
to control the lighting and acoustics of this high-end lounge.
100% interior Sylvia Leydecker,
Rems-Murr Hospital, Schorndorf,
Germany

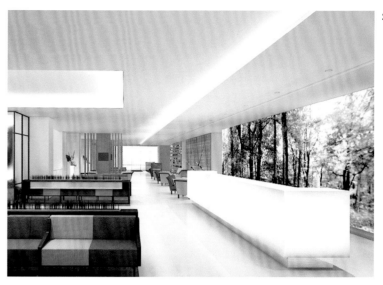

28

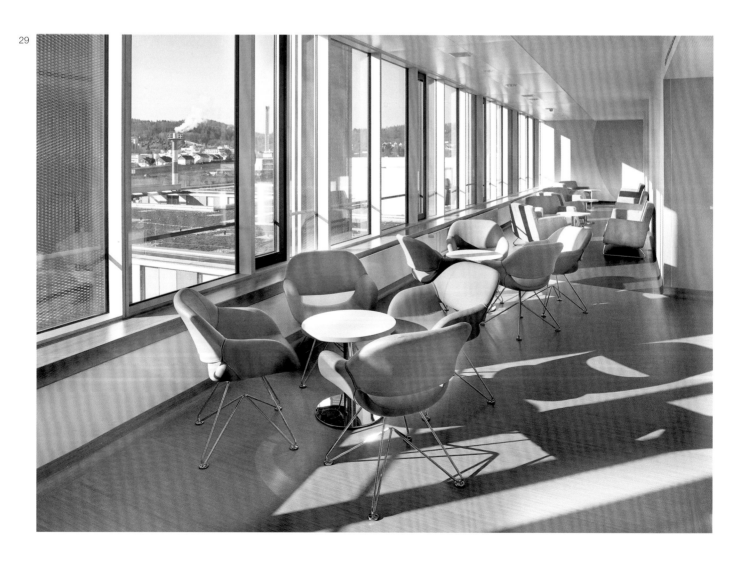

29

them, as well as safety mechanisms. The benefits are numerous, especially for comfort, energy-efficiency and cost savings. Equipment will notify the in-house facility management system when maintenance is necessary. Technical and practical support for patients can be partially provided by robots, as is already the case for example in some wards in San Francisco near Silicon Valley. Finally, smart applications can be used to create user and use profiles of patients and of staff with which both behavioural patterns and work routines can be optimised for the benefit of everyone.

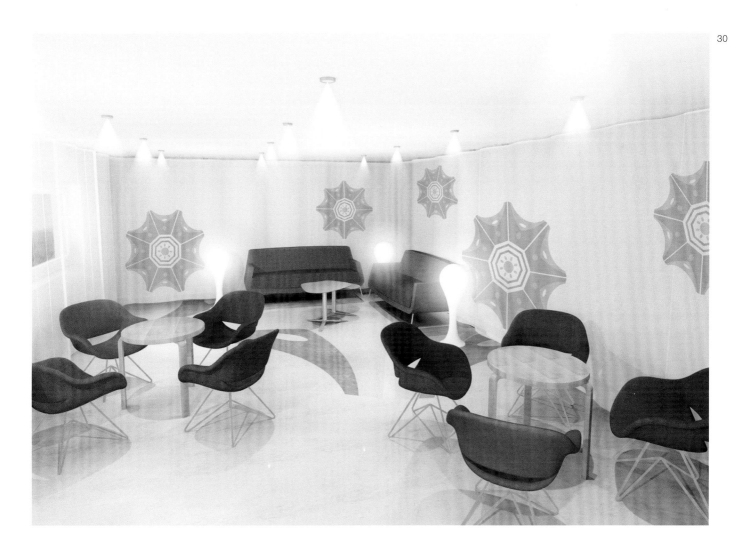

30

Designing a
salutogenic hospital
and patient's room

Alan Dilani

Research on salutogenesis highlights the role that architecture can play in patient recovery through environments that stimulate health and well-being. Salutogenic design principles create environments that support the well-being of patients as well as staff. The goal is to provide appropriate medical services in a stimulating environment that supports the healing process and is also creating an enjoyable and efficient workplace for the staff.

Adopting a salutogenic approach involves creatively and innovatively synthesising knowledge and expertise from multiple disciplines, including architecture, medicine, public health, psychology, design and engineering as well as culture, art and music. Salutogenic design focusses on positive psychosocial factors that reduce anxiety and strengthen an individual's sense of self by encouraging them to engage mentally and socially with their environment. A pleasant and enjoyable environment that captures the imagination of patients and visitors and encourages interaction has a positive psychological effect that minimises the anxiety patients often feel in unfamiliar and medical-centric hospital environments.

The International Academy for Design & Health has undertaken extensive empirical research into the salutogenic design of healthcare buildings, and studied hundreds of articles and literature related to the physical environment, health and behaviour to identify and explain the benefits of psychosocially supportive design and the power of salutogenic design spaces to influence health and well-being.

A salutogenic
patient's room

A patient's room should be designed to accommodate the needs of people of all ages and sizes and be designed as welcoming and engaging spaces for all users, particularly in communal spaces where patients and their families come together.

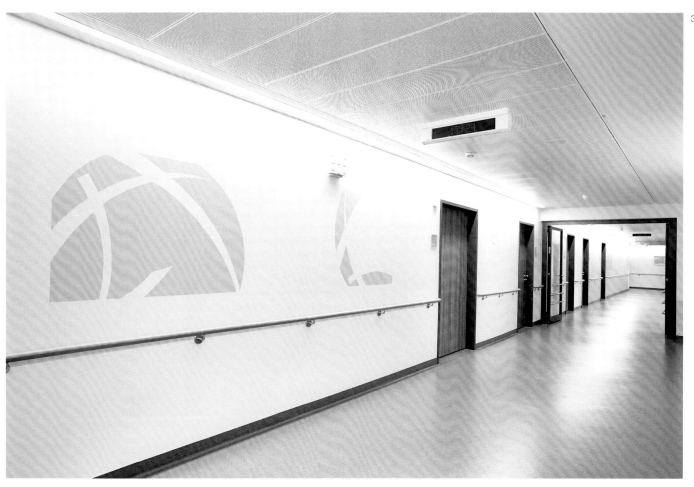

31

At Melbourne Royal Children's Hospital, the patient rooms are designed as safe and pleasant interiors that look directly onto an adjacent park and offer a view of the sky which can be seen from the bed. Parents and/or carers can stay the night on a visitor's bed in the same room. Contact to the natural environment through the window contributes to the recovery of the patient.

Art not only helps to make spaces more attractive; it also acts as a positive distraction during examination and treatment. The decoration of the walls of the Royal Children's Hospital use imagery that is both beautiful and educational, reflecting the nature of Australia. The images have thematic relevance to the focal areas of the hospital. In treatment rooms, this form of positive distraction creates stimulation and gives patients a sense of control so that they feel less vulnerable and more relaxed and comfortable with the procedure. Artwork is creative and stimulating. It evokes sensations that are life-affirming and creates a sense of well-being for both patients and visitors. For staff too, artwork acts as a positive intellectual stimulus. The salutogenic design of patient rooms focusses therefore on creating environments that minimise the causes of stress and help patients to better manage the level of stress associated with disease and hospitalisation.

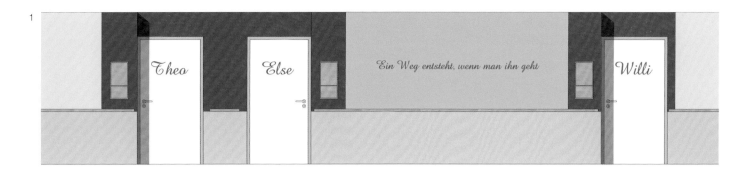

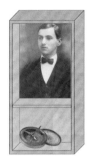 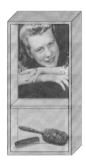 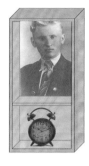

1 Reminiscence therapy is the principle behind this wall design. 100% interior Sylvia Leydecker, Maria-Hilf Hospital, Brilon, Germany

2 People with dementia often recognise stars from times past, helping them have a more positive attitude. Maria-Hilf Hospital

3 An earth-coloured floor creates a sense of stability. Warm colours dispel any impression of sterility and contribute to the residents' well-being. Maria-Hilf Hospital

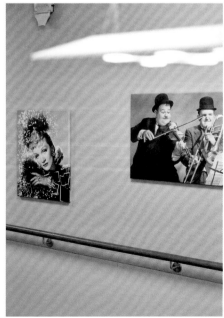 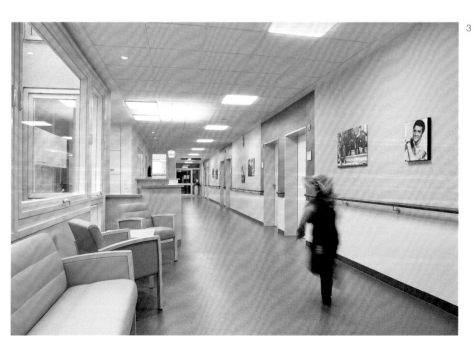

Old age and dementia

Demographic trends in many of the world's industrialised nations, among them Japan and Germany, require designers to give serious thought to the design of environments for an ever-aging society. The number of elderly patients is expected to rise dramatically in the coming years. Population figures show a proportionately greater increase in older people who will still be active, and indeed healthy, for several years to come but sooner or later will need to go to hospital and may become dependent on care. Even then, not everyone will follow precisely this pattern as people age differently. Patients with dementia or cognitive impairments are especially demanding for hospitals and staff, not just with respect to the individual attention each patient requires but also the comparatively long period of residence.

These developments have led to the setting-up of geriatric wards in many hospitals in recent years. A complicating factor in geriatric wards is the aspect of multi-morbidity among older patients.

This means that patients have multiple physical impairments alongside the primary complaint; for example, they may find it difficult to walk and also do not see or hear well. Conditions such as diabetes, incontinence, gout or rheumatism are further common examples.

Reducing potential dangers in patient rooms

Vision impairments most commonly cause orientation problems. In old age, not only does one's ability to see clearly diminish but also the ability to register colours. Clarity is a major help, for example large type against a contrasting background, or a seat colour that can be seen clearly against its context. Floors polished to a reflective surface are disconcerting to those who feel uncertain when walking and can even result in dramatic falls. Trip hazards should be avoided, both real and perceived: a slight change in floor level may not be noticed; or a change in floor material may be mistaken for a step. Typical situations are material changes that mark different areas, inlays or transitions between spaces. Blue floor coverings are sometimes used intentionally to limit the wandering tendency of dementia sufferers, who mistakenly perceive the blue as water, and therefore as a barrier. Doors and reveals that blend tone-in-tone with the wall may not be noticed by people with impaired vision, in effect serving as a simple form of camouflage. Both methods can be used to discourage patients from entering areas the hospital does not wish them to be in. The same principle applies to staircases and rooms for ancillary functions.

Rooms should be evenly illuminated to avoid both glare and hard shadows that people with poor sight many find hard to interpret. Trailing cables are typical trip hazards, not just for old people. Furniture must be stable and not topple over when a patient leans on it or holds onto it while getting up or sitting down. For this group

of patients, a fall in hospital can often have far-reaching consequences. Broken bones are to be expected and may lead to lengthy complications or worse. The liability risks that hospitals face are also considerable, and, in most cases, avoidable. The design of dementia-friendly environments can both improve the geriatric patients' sense of well-being and reduce behavioural difficulties.

Dementia patients often have orientation difficulties, which can be tackled by design means. The provision of clear points of orientation, such as a clock, sofa or bench placed at a strategic point, can help people know where they are heading or cause them to turn back. Distinct items placed at key points act as visual cues and memory markers, and avoid the disorientating effect of bland environments. This, together with the creation of circular routes, helps dementia patients follow their urge to move without getting lost. In some cases, these have since been replaced with simpler, straight pathways to avoid the risk of dehydration.

4

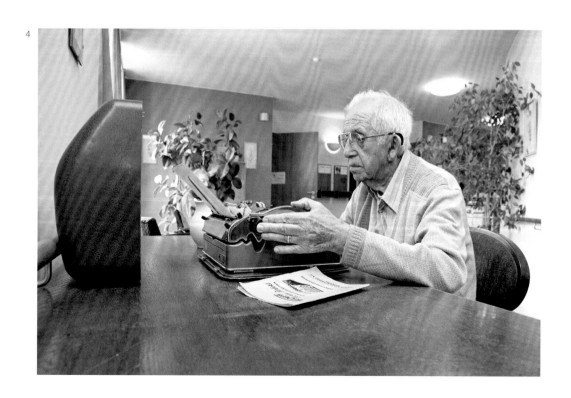

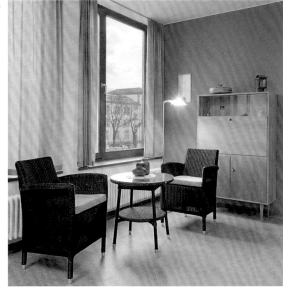

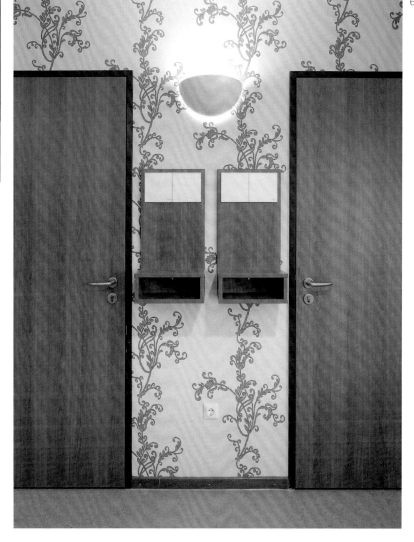

4 The elderly retain their compe-
tencies. Feddersen Architekten,
Dementia Competence Centre,
Nuremberg, Germany

5 A homely sitting area with individual
furniture. Dementia Competence
Centre

6 Personalisable door entry areas
help provide orientation. Dementia
Competence Centre

The course of the day also provides orientation. A structured daily routine that reflects the progression of the patients' day rather than the time plan of the staff contributes to their quality of life. Circadian lighting can be employed as a cue to influence the patients' biorhythms and their sleep-wake cycles.

Bathroom

The arrangement of sanitaryware in the bathroom should ensure that the WC can be seen immediately on opening the door, so that patients cannot overlook it and fail to go to the toilet. To facilitate a safe stay in hospital, bathrooms should be evenly illuminated without strong shadows, and be equipped with sufficient handrails and supports in a clearly visible, contrasting colour, along with a shower stool and floor-flush shower tray with anti-slip coating.

Reminiscence therapy through design

Reminiscence therapy has proven an effective way of activating the existing potential and competencies of dementia patients: objects from the person's own biography, whether photos of stars from the past or home furnishings such as an old-fashioned record player, sofa, living room standard lamp or favourite tablecloth can be incorporated to help activate memories. Similar effects can be achieved with spaces that cater for a long-submerged talent such as a love of painting, a passion for playing the piano or a talent for dancing. Memories are not only visual but are also triggered by other senses such as hearing.

This biographical potential is presently only rarely considered in the design of patient rooms, where heavy, ornate, traditional furnishings still seem to predominate. People who have lived other ways of life, for example in a modern, Bauhaus-inspired, design-conscious house, are better served by more open rooms with clean lines, unadorned sur-

faces and Bauhaus furniture. In other biographies, art or pop-art may feature strongly, or a Woodstock atmosphere with patchwork quilts, multi-coloured sculptures and lava lamps of the kind normally seen in "snoezelen rooms". Other elderly people may prefer a sense of casual noblesse reminiscent of Christian Dior and French chic. Each person has their own respective background and patient room design for the elderly should incorporate more possibilities for variation.

Multi-sensory design

Multi-sensory perception plays an important role for people with dementia due to their heightened emotional response. Pleasant fragrances can add to a sense of well-being, while the smell of food can be used to encourage people to eat regularly. Discreet music from the "good old days" likewise creates a sense of familiarity and well-being. All these can help patients and residents forget the hospital context. While it cannot necessarily prevent improper or even aggressive behaviour, it can reduce its incidence.

Colours and patterns

Floors in earthy colours communicate a sense of reassuring solidity. A reflective, polished floor, by contrast, can make people feel unsteady and put them at risk of slipping, regardless of colour. Blue floors can sometimes be mistaken for water. Yellow tones, accentuated with terracotta and apricot, create warm, comforting interiors; however, their use in patient rooms for older people has become somewhat ubiquitous. A balanced mix of pleasant sand and beige tones in combination with an off-white can be more effective. Terracotta ad infinitum can be counter-productive as pastel tones need accent colours to avoid becoming monotonous. Harmonious colour combinations together with the judicious use of accents according to a coherent overall design concept are the primary components of a convincing design concept.

7 A record player in the sitting room appeals to the sense of hearing and generally elevates the spirits. 100% interior Sylvia Leydecker, Maria-Hilf Hospital, Brilon, Germany

8 A functional bathroom in a geriatric ward with a pleasant colour concept. Maria-Hilf Hospital

9 Colour and material collage for a geriatric ward. Maria-Hilf Hospital

10 The attractive patina of an external wall in real life. Everything and everyone ages.

7
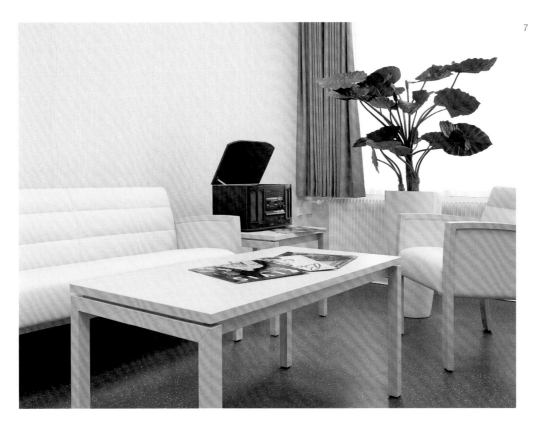

8
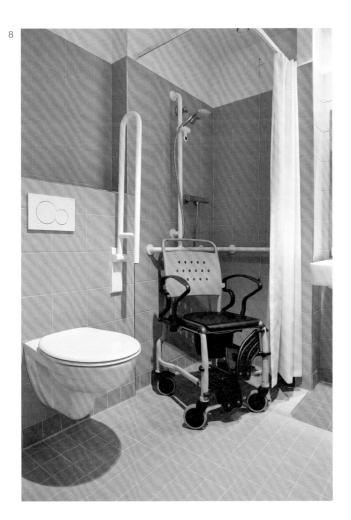

9
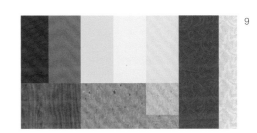

10
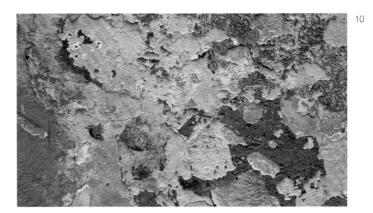

Patterns originate from and evoke different contexts and epochs: baroque sumptuousness, striped clarity, floral nature, dramatic photography or alternatively motifs from the Biedermeier period, from Art Nouveau, Bauhaus, hippy culture or the patterns of the Memphis Group from Milan. Discreet patterns create a homely impression and can be practical, for example for seating upholstery. Large-format patterns on wallpaper or curtains, on the other hand, may cause anxiety as they can be mistakenly interpreted as menacing figures by people with dementia. Textiles in general create a homely impression and have a pleasant haptic feel that signals quality of life. All textiles must, however, be functional, i.e. conform to fire safety requirements, be resistant to soiling and staining, be easy to clean, resistant to urine and able to withstand cleaning with disinfectants.

In terms of haptic qualities, handrails are especially important. Wood is warm to the touch, unlike steel, especially for patients with gout or rheumatism.

Handles and furniture knobs should be easy to grip, for example with a bow or D-handle so that patients can hook their fingers behind them to pull.

Sensors

Many digital devices now exist as useful aids for hospital use, for example carpets with sensors that register if someone has fallen over, or RFID sensors that signal when patients attempt to leave a ward. Sensors make it possible to regulate door entry and room functions such as light levels and room temperature. Last but not least, they also monitor the patient in bed. Telemedicine, vital signs monitoring and digital patient records will soon play an increasingly important role, as will care robots that will replace staff for certain functions. In San Francisco for example, robots are already in use in some patient wards, where tech giants such as Google, Facebook and similar

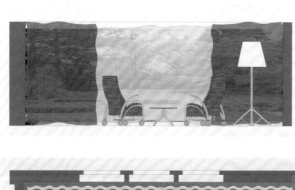

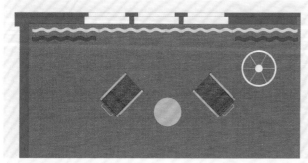

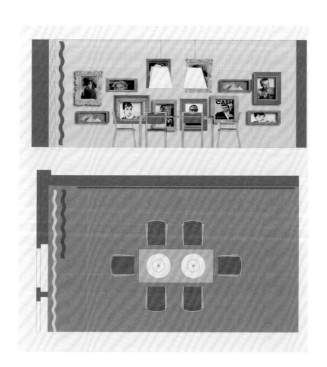

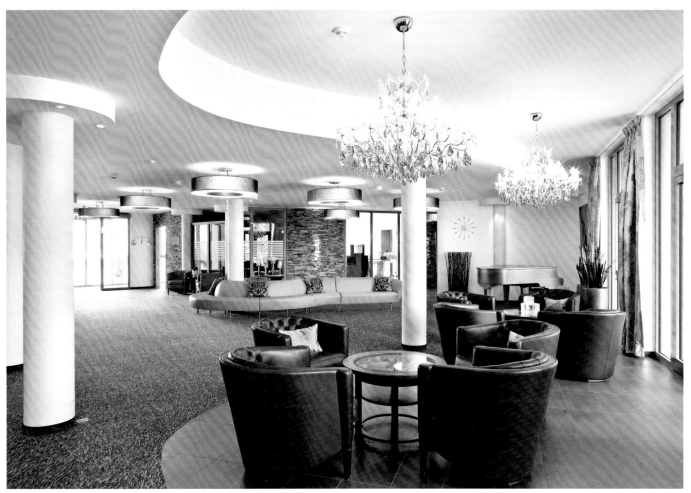

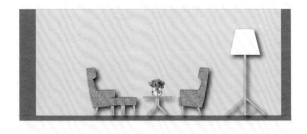

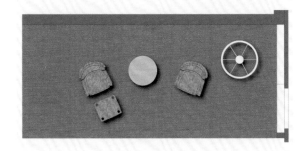

11 Layouts of different living areas.
    100% interior Sylvia Leydecker,
    Alexianer Geriatric care, Berlin,
    Germany

12 The forms, colour concept,
    materials and lighting of this
    assisted living centre contribute
    to the high quality of the interior.
    100% interior Sylvia Leydecker,
    Wohnen am Kurhaus, Hennef,
    Germany

13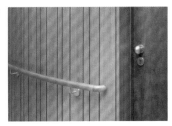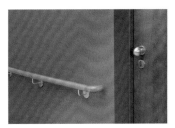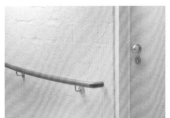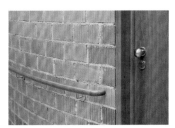

13 Wooden handrails are warm to the touch, regardless of the wall material. Feddersen Architekten, Dementia Competence Centre, Nuremberg, Germany

14 Corridor with a modern design. [s]innenarchitektur, Ansbach District Clinic, Germany

15 Bathroom for patients who need assistance during bathing. 100% interior Sylvia Leydecker, Hospice of the Foundation Marien Hospital, Euskirchen, Germany

14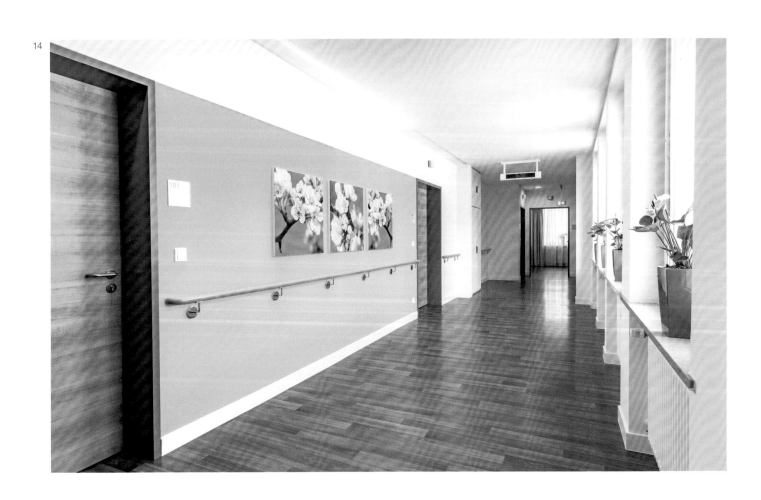

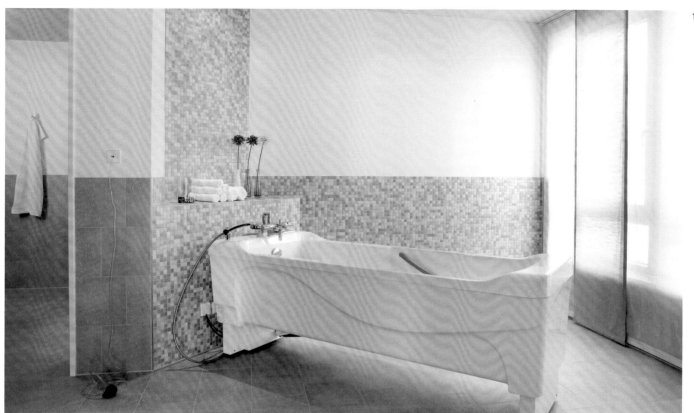

companies are spearheading their development. It is through their pioneering research and development work that such advances have become possible. Cultural characteristics also play a role: some cultures, such as Japan's "Manga culture" are more open to the use of technology in everyday life.

It is a fact that the number of older patients will increase overall and facilities will need to respond accordingly. Older people need particular care and attention, and in some cases are even completely helpless. At some point, they will inevitably find themselves going in and out of care facilities and hospitals. The design of patient rooms not only as practical and tolerable spaces but as appropriate, good-quality living environments is therefore a matter of ensuring human dignity.

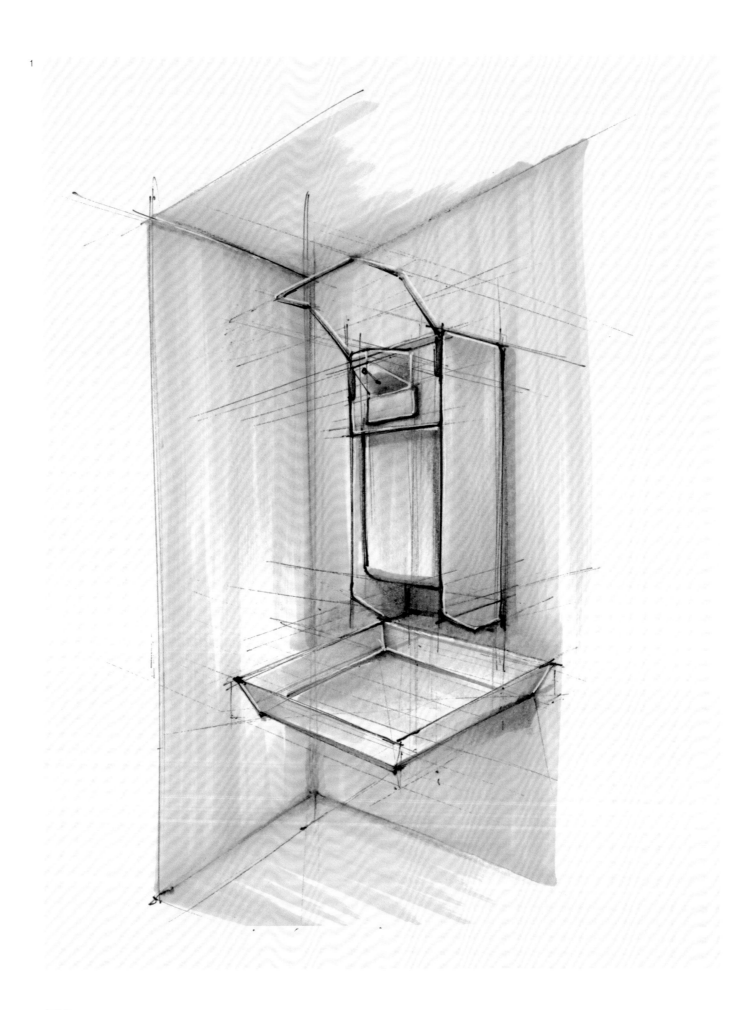

Ensuring hygiene

Patient rooms are first and foremost safe environments for patients while they recover, and hygiene plays a vital role in this. In the prevention of nosocomial infections (NI) – infections contracted in healthcare environments – most attention is given to hand hygiene, followed by the room environment and cleaning. Preventing the transmission of pathogenic bacteria and germs is nevertheless a factor of the hygienic conditions of the room, which is influenced by the design of the (interior) architecture. Contact with even minute levels of diarrhoea-inducing viruses or bacteria, such as the Norovirus or EHEC, on contaminated surfaces is sufficient to become infected.

The design of hospital patient rooms must therefore be part of a broader strategy to prevent the transmission of such infections. In Germany, the recommendations of the Commission for Hospital Hygiene and Infection Prevention (KRINKO) at the Robert Koch Institute (RKI) and the guidelines of the German Society for Hospital Hygiene (DGKH) set out hygiene requirements for the functional design and construction of rooms in hospitals. Like the DGKH, the Canadian Community and Hospital Infection Control Association (CHICA) also recommends increasing the proportion of single rooms, at least in new buildings, as a basic means of improving hygiene. In the USA, the new Safety Risk Assessment (SRA) Toolkit developed by the Center for Health Design (CHD) provides information on improving patient safety. Several other organisations also provide relevant information, including the Healthcare Infection Control Practices Advisory Committee (HICPAC), the Centers for Disease Control and Prevention (CDC), the Environmental Health Services (EHS), the National Center for Environmental Health (NCEH) or the Center for

Environmental Health (CEH). The phenomenon of hospitalism, resulting from infections contracted in hospital through contact with infected blankets and similar items, was in the past quite widespread. Today, hospitals do their utmost to combat hospital-acquired methicillin-resistant staphylococcus aureus (HA-MRSA) bacteria.

The dramatic rise in resistant germs in general gives cause for concern, especially when traditional means such as antibiotics are no longer effective. On the other hand, statistics in recent years show a slight downward trend. Nosocomial infections are not uncommon and the alarming number of more than 20,000 cases of death per year in the EU alone and several hundred thousand around the world every year (the statistics vary) are reason enough to devote considerable attention to hygiene concerns. Healthcare-associated infections (HAI) are a problem all over the world, and must therefore always be considered in the context of the built environment.

Hospital patients are inevitably more susceptible to contracting infections as their immune system is weakened by their illness. This applies to patients with injuries too, even when their general constitution is good. The World Health Organisation's global campaigns "Clean Care is Safer Care" and "Save Lives: Clean Your Hands", launched in 2005, as well

2 Matching hygienic modular seating and play elements in pediatric practice. 100% interior Sylvia Leydecker, waiting room In a paediatric practice, Dres. Schumann-Winckler-Schumann, Cologne, Germany

3 A visibly clean surface in a toilet. 100% interior Sylvia Leydecker, Hospice of the Foundation Marien Hospital, Euskirchen, Germany

4–5 Designs for a functional but also emotionally pleasing patient room in a rehabilitation clinic: variants with "BlueSKY" and "YellowSUN" atmospheres. 100% interior Sylvia Leydecker, Dr. Becker Rhein-Sieg Clinic, Nümbrecht, Germany

3

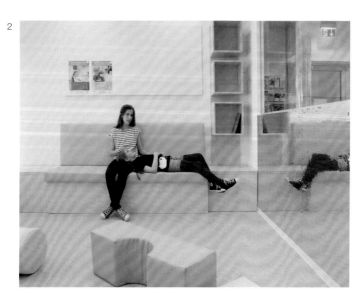

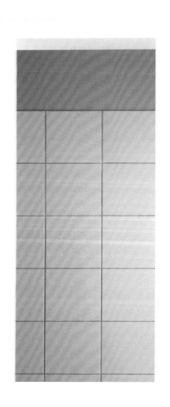

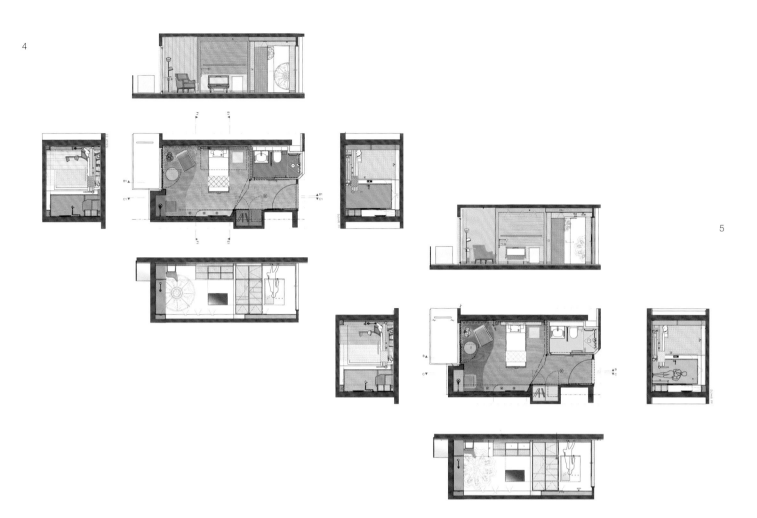

as the German "Aktion Saubere Hände" campaign, which is based on the WHO campaigns, show how necessary hand hygiene is at the right time and in the right way, and how important it is to have information about it (the publication "A report on the June 2015 – January 2016 WHO global Hand Hygiene Self-Assessment Framework survey" is worth reading in this context). The campaigns highlighted the role of cleaning one's hands and the benefit of placing not just one but several hand disinfectant dispensers around a room, ideally with a drip pan to prevent disinfectant damaging the floor.

The interior design of environments for patients as part of a prevention strategy for avoiding nosocomial infections requires the planning of hygienic surfaces and construction details that are not only easy to clean when first installed, but also remain easy to clean for a long time to come. Well-designed construction detailing, for example a cove junction between floor and wall, is of little use when poorly executed or when it becomes defective after a short while. Careful, forward-thinking detailing can help avoid risks that may arise, for example, out of a desire to save costs.

Surfaces in hospitals must still fulfil their functional requirements, especially with regard to hygiene, irrespective of how old they are. Upholstery materials, for example, must be easy to clean, urine-resistant and able to withstand wet cleaning with disinfectants. Products that are designed for hospital use tend to be the better choice because they have special upholstery seams, construction joints, screw fixings and materials made explicitly for better hygiene and cleaning.

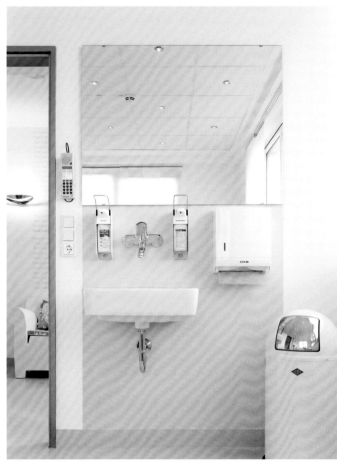

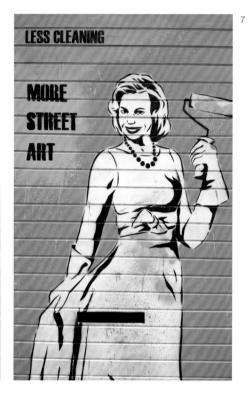

Beds are in direct contact with patients, have sensor-controlled electrical and mechanical parts, and are even classed as medical products. All parts need to be disinfected and should therefore not have gaps that are hard to reach and clean. Gaps are generally problematic for cleaning and hygiene, for example between floorboards and tiles, hence the predominance of strip materials such as linoleum or vinyl, or the use of large-format tiles that have fewer joints.

A few manufacturers have collaborated to combine different products in a single, optimised system: door manufacturers, and material and door handle producers, for example, have joined forces to create germ-free door solutions for hygienically sensitive areas. These systems act as an effective and lasting barrier to germ transmission.

Anti-bacterial surfaces, such as those of specially-coated door handles, high-pressure laminate (HPL) panels or anti-bacterial varnishes should be reserved for use in healthcare environments, partly in response to the problem of resistance development but also because it is here that they are most useful in fulfilling hygiene requirements and ensure hygiene in general. Products that exhibit certain surface characteristics in laboratory testing may not behave the same way in practice. Testing methods should therefore reflect real conditions and be related to individual cases to obtain a better idea of the paths of infection and associated risks, instead of using standard laboratory approaches, as is the Japanese way. Japanese standards employ petri dishes in which the test material is studied under moist and warm conditions. While these parameters may be ideal conditions for germs, they never exist

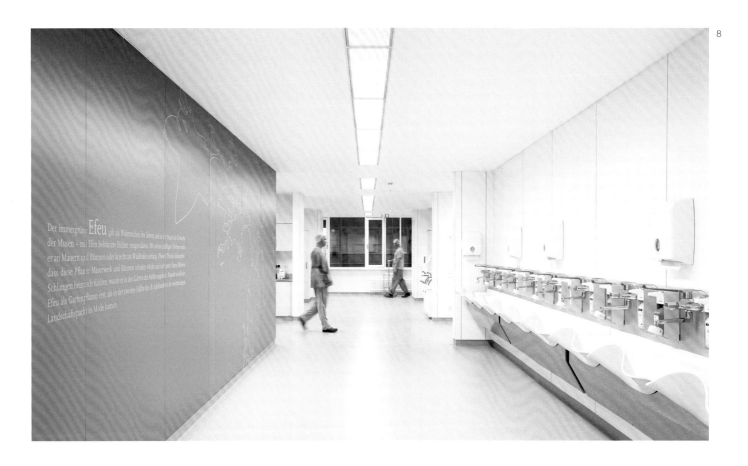

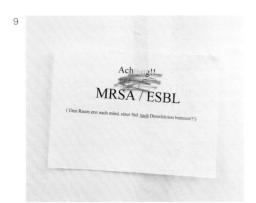

8

9

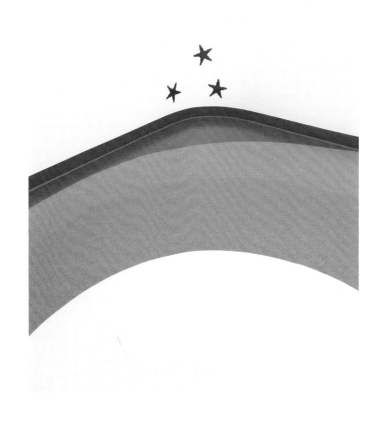

6   Clean and simple but also perfectly hygienic.
100% interior Sylvia Leydecker,
Obstetrics Unit, Maria-Hilf Clinic, Brilon, Germany

7   Not all contexts take hygiene as seriously as the
healthcare sector.

8   Disinfection is paramount in operating theatres.
a|sh architekten, Siloah-Oststadt-Heidehaus
Clinic, Hanover, Germany

9   "MRSA/ESBL Disinfection. Wait at least an hour
before re-entering the room" – such notices
should in future no longer be necessary.

10   Hygienic and stylish – a rounded corner
to a room. 100% interior Sylvia Leydecker,
Stammen dental surgery, Grevenbroich, Germany

in practice on the surface of a door handle. One way or the other, anti-bacterial, hygienic surfaces cannot replace effective cleaning and disinfection and do not obviate the need to observe hygiene regulations. Potential carriers of infection, such as staff uniforms, need to be identified and suitable measures devised block the path of transmission.

The cleaning and disinfection of surrounding areas and surfaces is likewise fundamental to reducing the transmission of infection and should feature in hygiene plans. Wiping and cleaning surfaces such as floors, doors and furniture is different to disinfecting beds and textiles. The former is undertaken by ward cleaning staff, while the latter is undertaken by machinery in the hospital laundry. Textiles such as curtains, for example, are laundered at high temperatures and subsequently disinfected. Dirt and bacterial contamination mostly concerns door handles, switches and touch panels, telephones and bedding and bed linen. Surfaces that are within reach of the patient are especially important in terms of hygiene. Touch-less fittings and doors that are sensor-operated can be advisable in such cases.

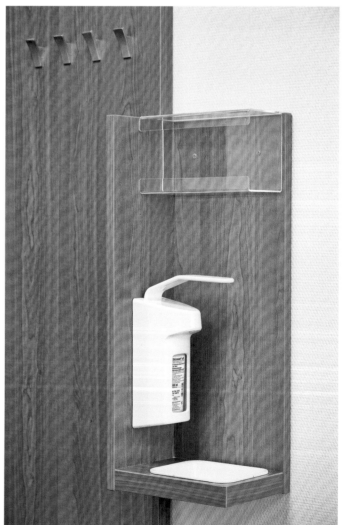

12

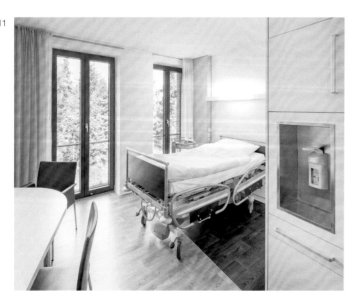

11

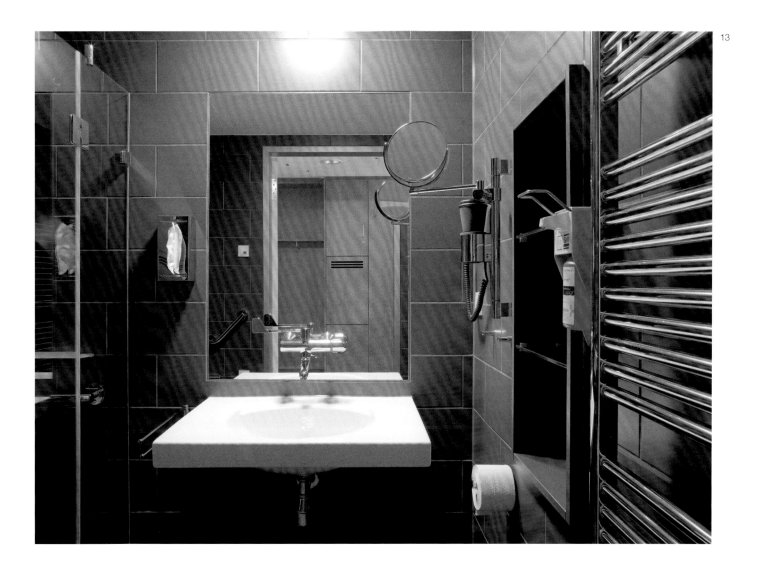

11 A disinfectant dispenser integrated into
    the furnishings. GSP Gerlach Schneider
    Partner Architekten, confort ward,
    Ammerhand-Clinic, Westerstede,
    Germany

12 A disinfectant dispenser integrated into
    the furnishings. 100% interior Sylvia
    Leydecker, Rems-Murr Hospital,
    Winnenden, Germany

13 Dark bathroom designs can be just as
    hygienic. 100% interior Sylvia
    Leydecker, Sana Clinics, Bad Wildbad,
    Germany

14 Careful detailing and construction is
    important to ensure maximum hygiene.

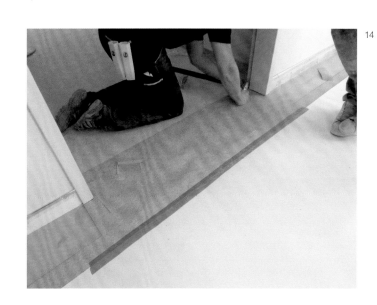

The focus is therefore not just on visual cleanliness but on interrupting the path of infection transmission and preventing re-colonisation of bacteria. Visible damage to surfaces and other areas where dirt can collect should not be tolerated: for germs, a minor crack or dent is the equivalent of a crater. In terms of cleanliness, matt surfaces on which wipe marks remain are just as problematic as uniformly-coloured floor surfaces that show every bit of dirt.

Microbial contamination is invisible: what looks clean can still be contaminated. The actual degree of contamination, whether of objects or people, can be determined using paddle testers, a method also used in medicine. Random sampling gives an overall impression of the degree of hygiene. A widespread problem is that cost-cutting limits the time available for cleaning, affecting the quality of cleaning.

Hygiene in hospitals is therefore about protecting people's health and can be promoted through the interior design of the patient's environment, and its surfaces and construction. While hygiene is paramount, it must also be balanced against the need to create a comfortable atmosphere conducive to recovery. Washable, sterile rubber cells will not help people recover. A feel-good atmosphere and hygiene are not mutually exclusive, and can and should ideally complement one another so that each has maximum benefit for the well-being of the patient.

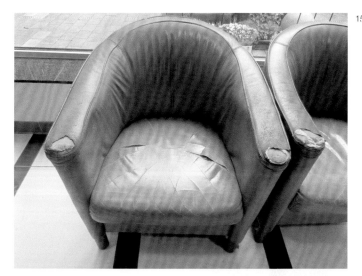

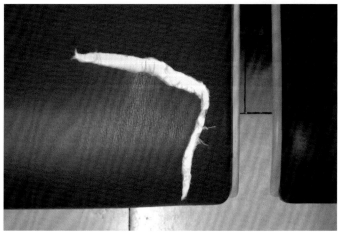

15 Worn and torn upholstery in hospital environments presents a hygiene risk.

16 Sometimes existing hygienic surfaces may be damaged.

17 Comfort for privately health-insured patients means disinfectant-resistant, fire-resistant, urine-impervious and, last but not least, comfortable and attractive furnishings. 100% interior Sylvia Leydecker, Rems-Murr Hospital, Winnenden, Germany

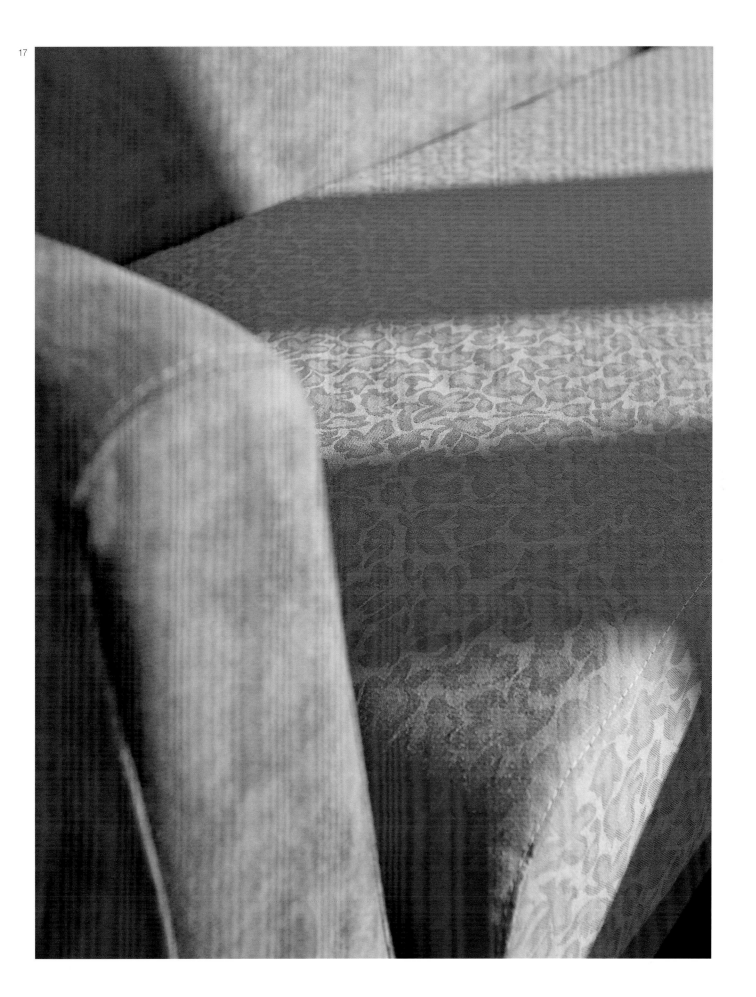

Hygiene and design in medical environments

Georg Daeschlein

18 Hygiene is indispensable in healthcare. 100% interior Sylvia Leydecker, FutureCare 2010, CeBIT, Hanover, Germany

18

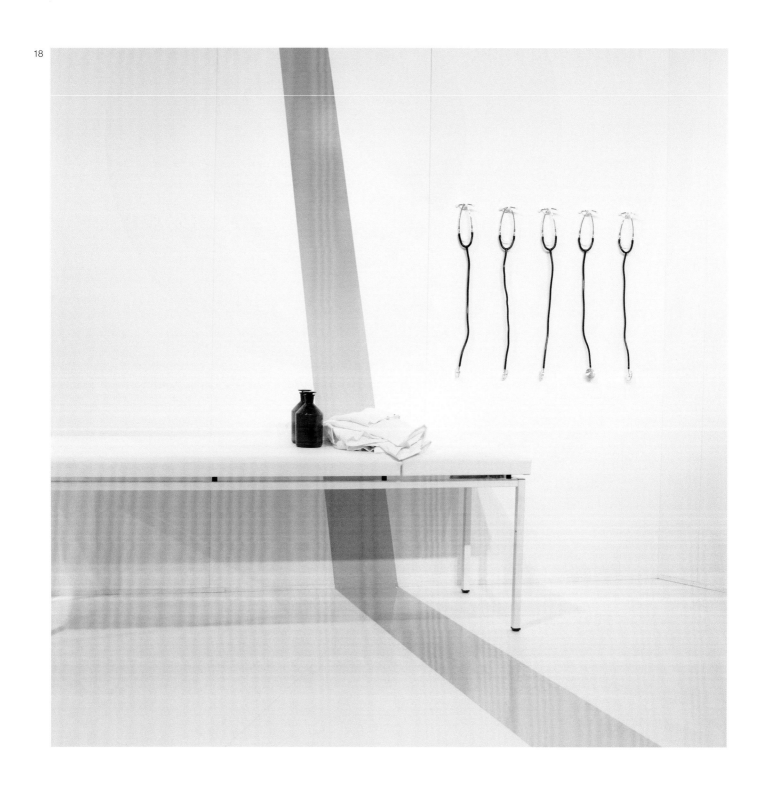

Visions for the patient room of the future and the hospital of the future have shifted significantly in recent years. One central aspect in this respect is the creation of atmospheres that promote and support the process of recovery. Current research shows that this has a more beneficial effect on the outcome of therapy than previously thought. Equally relevant is the role of positive feedback on the part of the staff, who will work more effectively in an environment that provides the best possible conditions for doing their job. One of the main reasons why it has taken so long – decades, in fact – to reach this conclusion, is the persistent belief that it is impossible to combine the demands of comfort and hygiene. The "zero tolerance" policy toward all surfaces that can potentially harbour germs has meant that generations of patients (and medical staff) have had to tolerate "sterile" space-station-style interiors that were often anything but as hygienic as they purported to be. At the time, these interiors were modelled on the hygienically clean interiors of industrial fabrication plants and laboratories. It's not hard to understand why: an environment that has few (contaminable) surfaces and reduces all necessary technical surfaces (machines, computers and other equipment) to an (industrially compatible) minimum, will offer optimum hygienic conditions, with minimal contamination and germ transmission, partly because there are fewer exposed surfaces and partly because these surfaces, whether floor, work surfaces or equipment surfaces, are quick and effective to hygienically disinfect. In addition such rooms should be well lit and minimise the number of visitors, as key potential carriers of bacteria in all parts of a hospital. It should also be obvious that the still common practice of modelling the design of patient rooms on high-security microbiological units of the kind seen in silicon chip or pharmaceuticals production facilities (as well as in many intensive care wards around the world) is not able to address the needs of people living with possibly life-threatening illnesses because it does not accommodate aspects of everyday life, instead reducing everything non-medical to the minimum functionality of a "clean room". This is

where excessive focus on hygiene can become a problem. It is not by chance that the accessories of daily life, with which people surround themselves, create a personal atmosphere that is diametrically opposed to the industrial concept of the "clean room". Architecture has learned that a comfortable, homely atmosphere is important for patient recovery, that good working conditions improve staff satisfaction, and that architecture is about more than the rational, functional and hygienic concerns, which on their own lead to intolerable "clean room" atmospheres that may make patients sicker rather than healthier.

Following the gradual move away from the "spaceship architecture" of care facilities, and of intensive care wards in particular, focus has shifted to finding acceptable compromises between ensuring hygiene and creating appropriate interiors through the means of interior architecture. At the same time, future architects learn about the mechanisms by which microorganisms interact with modern surfaces and, therefore, how to identify important determining factors for potential risks as well as preventive measures. This shift informs both modern architecture and modern hospital hygiene, although the relevant subject matters are still not adequately represented in the schooling of either discipline. Successful solutions are, therefore, highly dependent on the respective expertise of the individual architects and hygienists, and how they work together.

There are several key areas in which the interior design solution must conform as best possible to the specific hygiene requirements of hospital buildings. It is important to note that while these risk areas are essential for patient safety, their design should nevertheless align with the overall design concept to avoid specific key aspects and their technical implementation from compromising the overall architectural intention. While the simplest approach to fulfilling the technical requirements would, without doubt, be a suitably functional building, its net effect is diminished through the dominant focus on its technical realisation, although this makes it more straightforward to realise. In this context, it is worth noting, by way of example, that high-tech environments can lead both to more user errors and more negligent practices, for example with respect to day-to-day hygiene, when such environments lack the necessary degree of comfort. This too confirms a central tenet: medicine alone does not heal people; it helps them to heal themselves. Intensive care is no different in this respect. The most important task in a hospital (and of its architecture) is to support this process to the best possible degree. Here, Brecht's assertion that "one can kill a man with a miserable house" can be applied to the medical context. The hospital as a "spaceship to nowhere" can be as debilitating as the most dreaded disease, even more so due to its synergistic effects.

While the hospital of the future cannot do without water, it can do almost entirely without washing facilities. Studies are currently revealing how serious water- or aerosol-borne hospital infections derive from such locations as showers, toilets and washbasins. Ever since it became known that wet rooms and washing facilities play a significant role as reservoirs for multi-drug-resistant bacteria, hospitals have been working to reduce, convert, technically perfect and even partially eradicate wet washing facilities to prevent the emission of bacteria. By way of example, washing one's hands has now become a minimal affair near the room entrance and wardrobe, and the large surgical scrub sinks, once the pride of every operating room, have now all but disappeared, replaced with discreet basins just large enough to catch droplets of antiseptic washing agents as hands are being disinfected. Instead of washing, one disinfects certain parts of the skin, and scrubbing down is now the exception. By the same token, washbasins are disappearing from patient rooms in intensive care wards. People now wash using disposable moist antiseptic cloths that feel like a flannel but don't transmit germs. Toilets are being converted to rimless, flush-efficient toilets, and shower heads and taps are being fitted with special hygiene-improving filters.

One cannot overestimate the importance of light for overcoming illness! Light is the very antithesis of illness; light symbolises life, darkness death. As the patient wavers between life and death, it is not yet clear how much artificial help will tip the balance in favour of life. The value of light is most dramatically evident when the patient wakes to see sunlight, even if for the last time. The design of hospitals as large separate pavilion buildings in the early 1930s, and again in the 1950s, not only helped prevent the spread of infections. Patients were cared and treated from one side and visited from the other. These light-filled interiors were a hygienic reality. Aside from the well-known capacity of the UV component of sunlight to combat microorganisms, daylight had the psychological effect of dispelling darkness. For more than a hundred years, the uplifting effect of the colour blue has been used in medicine. Its therapeutic effect can be seen in the "blue light showers" installed in parks in Dresden and Leipzig, Germany, and in the pure blue used by Yves Klein in many of his works. Aside from its elevating effect on well-being, this light is used in care homes to treat osteoporosis. In short, light and hygiene are inextricably linked and light makes all the difference for good hygiene. Sufficient light is therefore an imperative part of hospital design. Where natural light is unavailable, artificial light sources should be used to optimal effect for the benefit of both staff and patients. What is good for healthy people is many times more important for people who are ill: the more incapacitated a person is, the more desperate their situation, the more dependent they are on their environment as they are less able to influence it.

To return to the comparison with living. Today, it is not Brecht's "miserable" conditions that make people sick, but the danger of taking hygienic concerns too far: "sterilising" the atmosphere through an excessive focus on hygiene can itself make people sick.

To be successful, modern medicine requires modern architecture, and modern architecture requires innovative medicine and innovative thinking.

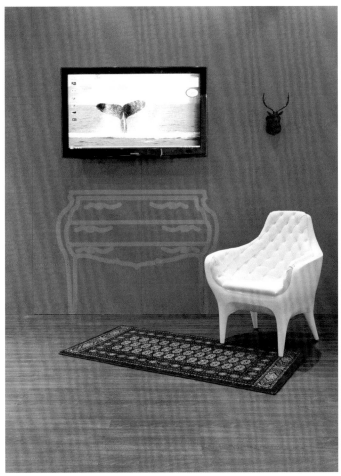

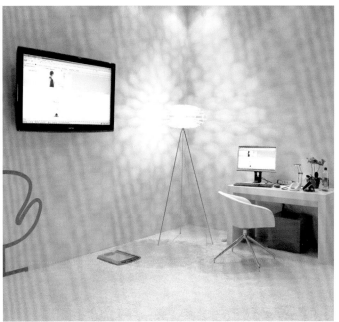

19–20 Digital media connects the home with the outside world without transmitting bacteria. Telemedicine systems such as Telehealth do the same for healthcare – irrespective of whether the user sits in a lifestyle-design interior or on a chintzy sofa. 100% interior Sylvia Leydecker, FutureCare 2009, CeBIT, Hanover, Germany

At present, however, the knowledge and understanding each discipline should have of the other is not part of the schooling of either profession. All too often it comes down to chance and circumstance: one medical facility moves into a freshly completed modern building, while another seems to be stuck in the last century. For this to change for the benefit of patients and of the nursing and medical staff who look after them, and not least to improve the practice of medicine in the respective society – those for whom these spaces are made and who will shape them in future, those for whom hygiene is but one, albeit essential, aspect – requires that both disciplines, architecture and medicine, broaden their horizons and open the bounds of their respective expertise to the needs and ultimate benefit of each other.

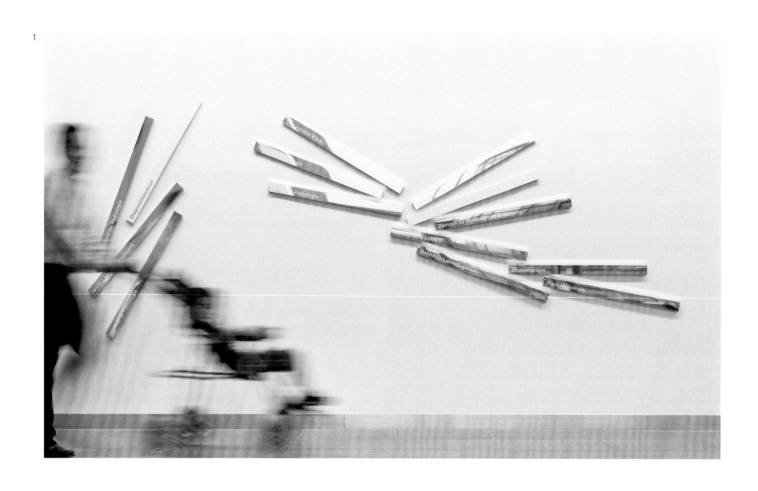

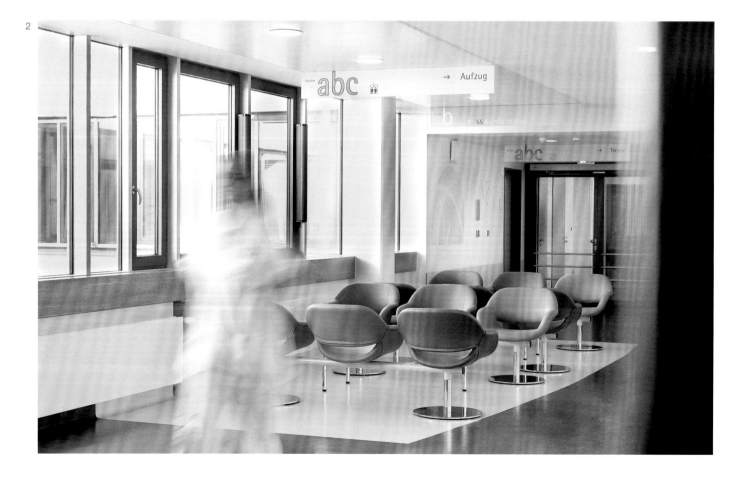

International developments and trends

1   The routes in modern hospitals
     lead in many directions. büro
     uebele visuelle kommunikation,
     Offenbach Clinic, Germany

2   An attractive, demarcated
     waiting area next to the lifts.
     100% interior Sylvia Leydecker,
     Rems-Murr Hospital,
     Winnenden, Germany

Healthcare is an issue of international dimensions. In our globalised world, it is necessary to coordinate international efforts in order to reduce health risks at a national level. Obvious examples include containing epidemics or the spread of MRSA bacteria, as well as developments such as the spread of tropical diseases in Europe due to climate change, as diseases do not stop at borders. It is therefore essential to think globally. At the same time, the cross-section of patients, and of staff, is becoming increasingly diverse and international. Migration around the world as well as international business travel and tourism have given rise to a mix of cultures, mentalities, languages and religions with different points of view and ways of life, as well as taboos and behavioural patterns. The design of healthcare environments must accommodate these different needs and reduce the potential for friction and conflicts. In addition, a good and financeable national health service is desirable that provides medical care for everyone, ideally with health-promoting interiors for all patients regardless of social status.

The need to consider polyethnic social demographics in the architectural and interior design of healthcare environments will become an increasingly important aspect of the design of interiors for patients. Architects and interior architects will need to consider this in the design of human-centred, safe and aesthetically attractive interiors, while also addressing economic and ecological considerations.

As mentioned in the introduction, structural conditions for healthcare vary around the world. Nevertheless, the projects shown in this book share a common theme: they focus on the needs of the patient and on environments that promote health and recovery. Ideally, they also reflect the healthcare providers' need for a tangible economic return, i.e. the operator's investment in design results in a billable service or quality level.

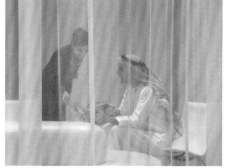

3

3 Arabian patient in discreet conversation. NBBJ, Dubai Mall Medical Center, United Arab Emirates

4 A calm atmosphere in a modern, forward-looking environment with lounge area and recessed TV. dwp, Jaypee Medical Centre, Noida, India

5 A hospital lobby that evokes the universe of the Native American culture. NBBJ, Chief Andrew Isaac Health Center, Fairbanks, Alaska, USA

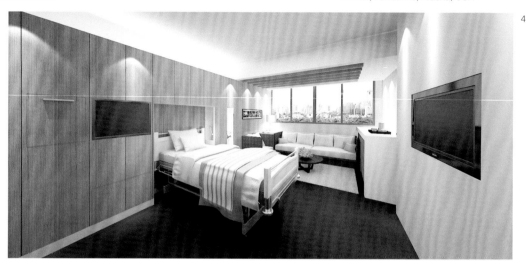

4

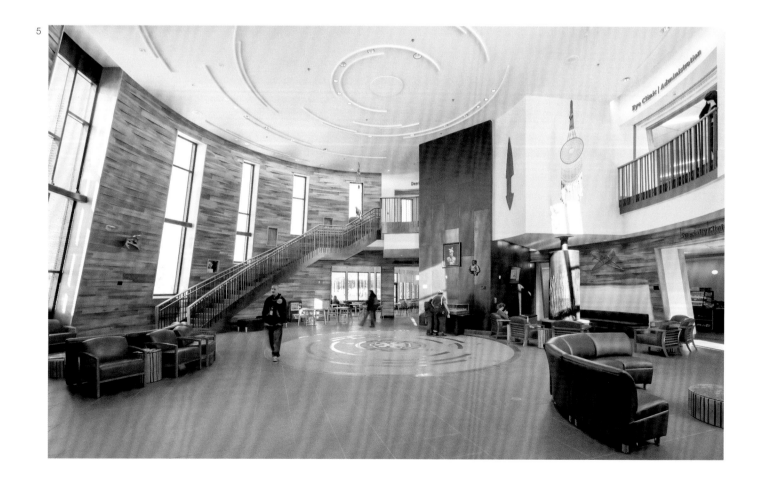

5

The following pages discuss some of the developments and trends currently gaining increasing importance around the world.

Medical tourism

Medical tourism – patients who travel elsewhere in the world to obtain the best possible modern medical treatment – is becoming increasingly popular among a growing group of affluent clients seeking special treatments such as cosmetic surgery, complex or specific health treatment or preventive medical measures. In many cases, patients are accompanied by relatives or even a small entourage of companions. Luxury, high-end healthcare providers compete with one another to attract this frequently wealthy clientele. Such healthcare environments are spacious and comfortable, with high-quality materials and bedding, excellent views and sometimes even a butler service, special culinary offerings and security guards to ensure privacy. The obvious discrepancy between this and the provision of "quality healthcare for everyone" can often be a balancing act for hospitals that provide both levels of service. Another facet of medical tourism is the increasing practice of travelling to a cheaper country, for example to Eastern Europe or Thailand, to receive medical care at more affordable rates.

Healing environments and Evidence-Based Design (EBD)

In the USA, significant advances have been made in the design of so-called healing environments that support a patient's process of recovery. Empirical research has shown that natural daylight, contact with nature and a pleasant indoor environment promote a sense of well-being that benefits patient recovery. Case studies and relevant topics have been scientifically studied and analysed to demon-

strate the benefit of such planning measures. The results confirm that Evidence-Based Design (EBD) serves as a useful planning tool in the design of healing environments. Through the study of patient environments, one can demonstrate how selected measures can benefit the process and speed of patient recovery, making the effect of design decisions measurable and verifiable. The related practice of salutogenic design likewise focusses on the well-being of the patient as its central principle.

Patient hotels

In some regions, such as Scandinavia, a combination of pragmatic reasons, increasing work pressures, and the need to reduce costs and improve patient comfort have led to the introduction of so-called patient hotels. The actual period spent in hospital is kept to a minimum, while the days prior to and after medical treatment, in which complex medical facilities (for example oxygen supply) and medical staff are not necessary, are spent in a less expensive room without special technical facilities, staffed by regular hotel personnel. This reduces costs considerably during the convalescing period. For a long time, this system seemed very promising for German hospitals. However, the different structure of healthcare in Germany – fewer local hospitals, longer travel distances for patients, as well as the specific billing modalities for private health insurers – means that this system is unworkable in Germany. For example, a shift in the proportion of single-bed rooms to multi-bed rooms within a hospital affects the billing scales for health services. This does not, however, contradict with a general desire for patient rooms with a more hotel-like atmosphere, which, on the contrary, is gaining increasing importance. Hotel chains around the world are already working together with hospitals to provide accommodation for relatives as well as for patients who need only specific medical services and can safely stay near to a hospital. In future, this may become more common, especially for preventive medical services provided by hospitals as outpatient services.

Psychosomatics

The always-on mentality of modern digital working patterns in industrialised nations such as Germany, Great Britain, Japan or the USA, along with concomitant stress and social isolation, has led to an increase in psychosomatic illnesses. The most common and now socially accepted manifestation of this is the so-called "burn out". The recovery period for psychosomatic illnesses is comparatively long compared with somatic illnesses, and nowadays affects all social classes and age groups. Psychosomatic clinics around the world are experiencing a rise in patient numbers, in turn resulting in the building of new facilities. Patients also typically stay for much longer – sometimes weeks or even months – and may return several times. In response to this, the design of patient rooms can offer possibilities for personalisation, for example through photos or other personal items. Patient environments should be open, transparent and life-affirming while also allowing patients to withdraw into an own safe environment as needed. Here, physical infirmity is less of an issue than mental well-being. The room design must therefore be particularly sensitive to the emotional state and needs of the patient and frequently need not cater for all the technical and functional requirements of a regular patient room. Here too, calm, restrained but also positive and life-affirming atmospheres are better than active spaces with an overload of stimuli.

Wellness

Wellness can significantly improve personal well-being, and is therefore also of benefit to patients. As a complement to medical care, it has developed into a flourishing global market.

Wellness interiors are high-quality environments designed for relaxation and prevention, with special focus on the sensory experience and pleasant atmospheres. Textures, fragrances, light, proximity to water and direct haptic experiences are some of the design means that architects and designers can use to corresponding effect. While medical competencies are invariably of primary importance in hospitals, the emotional needs of patients are increasingly being recognised: rooms that are peaceful and relaxing are typically most effective at supporting patient recovery, especially among anxious patients.

Healthcare for the elderly

Demographic transition has given renewed focus to the need for healthcare services tailored to the needs of the elderly. Countries such as Germany, France, Great Britain, the USA and Japan will need to provide additional facilities for elderly and aged patients, for example in the form of geriatric wards that can address the needs of patients with dementia or multiple physical disabilities. In addition, orthopaedic complaints are increasing significantly, especially among older patients, resulting in the need for hip or knee operations. Rehabilitation clinics will increasingly play a role, not just in healing but also in helping patients live a better life with a complaint. The industry has long identified more wealthy "silver agers" as a suitable target group for higher-quality offerings. Patient rooms tailored to the needs and desires of this predominantly younger group of elderly people follow the model of elegant high-class hotel rooms. Not all countries face this issue: countries such as Indonesia, where the average age is 30 years, will not need to address this aspect for many years to come.

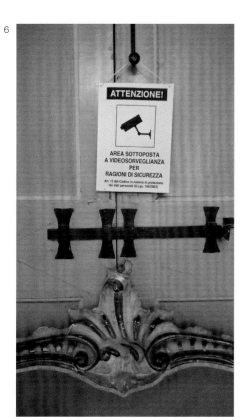

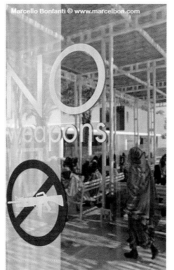

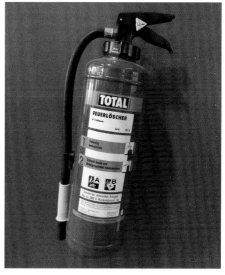

6	CCTV is seemingly every-where in the name of total security.		The Salam Centre for Cardiac Surgery, Khartoum, Sudan
7	In some countries, it is not obvious that weapons should not be taken into hospitals. TAMassociati,	8	Fire safety provisions also mean making fire extinguishers easy to find.

Universal Design

Universal Design means designing for usability by everyone and creating barrier-free access for everyone, regardless of ability or disability. Barrier-free access is often regarded as being synonymous with wheelchair accessibility, but it also means considering the needs of people with visual or hearing impairments as well as able-bodied people with pushchairs. The principle of "design for all" is fundamentally democratic, and is gradually being anchored in legislation in many parts of the world, especially for new public buildings. It is therefore an aspect that must be reflected – functionally and aesthetically – in the design of hospital interiors.

Rules and regulations

Regulations and standards governing the planning of healthcare interiors differ from country to country as there is no universally applicable regulatory framework. Regulations exist as a means for public authorities to assess the correct and safe execution of design and building work. Although the German building regulations for hospital buildings, the Krankenhausbauverordnung (KhBauVo), have been formally withdrawn in many Federal States to decrease bureaucracy, they have proven workable and are still used as a guideline in practice. Constructions correspond to standards that are different around the world, for example US or German standards.

Regulations governing functional aspects such as fire safety likewise differ from country to country, and even from state to state within a country, and can result in different planning stipulations, for example, for the width of corridors or doors. For example, ceiling-mounted lifts are used widely in France to assist in raising and lowering patients, but much less so in neighbouring countries. Floor coverings with a slip resistance rating of R10 are mandatory in Great Britain to prevent falls, but are not permissible in Germany as they do not fulfil

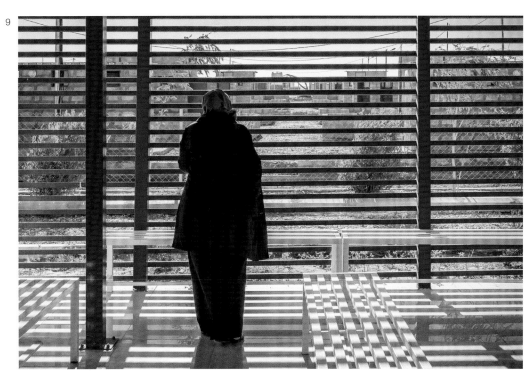

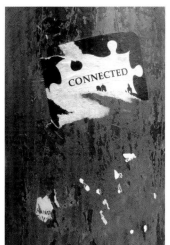

hygiene requirements. An exception is allowed only for the floors of wet rooms, for which special ratings exist (10a and 10b). Are people more susceptible to slipping in the British Isles than on the Continent? Are substances more prone to catching fire in Bavaria than at the North Sea coast? Reconciling fall prevention and hygiene requirements is, it would seem, an ongoing balancing act in the design of healthcare interiors. Whatever the outcomes of the various considerations are, the protection and safety of users must be paramount.

Technological advances

The use of the BIM methodology as a planning tool makes working internationally a reality by enabling different planning disciplines to work from different locations and at different times on the same project. The BIM methodology models projects in three dimensions rather than two and includes linked information such as time schedules and

costs. Data exchange interfaces between partners must, however, function reliably to avoid the risk of data loss and ensure data safety.

The processing of such vast quantities of data requires corresponding computer and server technology. This in turn increases the contribution of IT infrastructure to global carbon emissions, which is becoming an environmental problem of global scale. In addition, individual technological innovations in medical care provision, whether in diagnostics, operating theatres or telemedicine, will need to be networked into an overall system to be of long-term value. Digital developments also play a role in the design of patient rooms, not only for infotainment but also patient safety, for example using sensors or access control mechanisms. Digital comfort elements and control mechanisms are likewise part of the room design, as seen in the "hospital engineering lab" project by the Fraunhofer Institute for Software and Systems Engineering (ISST) in Duisburg, Germany. Compared to advances in digital technology, however,

9 A phone to one's ear is the
image of the modern digital world.
TAMassociati, Health Centre in
a refugee camp, Iraq

10 Everything is connected,
whether analogue or digital.

the incorporation of aesthetic and emotional aspects in the design of patient rooms still lags clearly behind.

Politics

Politics acts at different levels, for example EU-wide or at a national level, to define the boundary conditions for legislation. Organisations such as the World Health Organisation (WHO) or the United Nations (UN) influence politics at a global level. Examples include the WHO "Save Lives: Clean Your Hands" initiative, the WHO's call for reduced noise levels in intensive care units or the efforts of the UN to ensure clean drinking water for everyone, as a means of preventive healthcare. In the design of patient rooms, this affects aspects such as the placement of disinfectant dispensers. Political policy also affects the financing of healthcare systems, and in turn the expectations that individual patients have of their healthcare system.

Multi-cultural aspects

The multi-cultural nature of modern society, with people from diverse backgrounds and countries of origin, applies equally to patients and medical and healthcare staff. While not all hospitals are as culturally diverse, this aspect should not be ignored. Some societies, such as that of Singapore, are a mix of Western, Asian and Arabic cultures, while others have a dominant immigrant group, for example Turkish people in Germany, North Africans in France, Indians in Great Britain or Mexicans in parts of the USA. The intermixing of cultures is therefore just as evident in hospital operations. Irrespective of globalisation and internationalisation, the day-to-day operation of a hospital takes place locally.

The following projects serve as a source of inspiration and show selected examples that reflect the current state of the art and illustrate key developments.

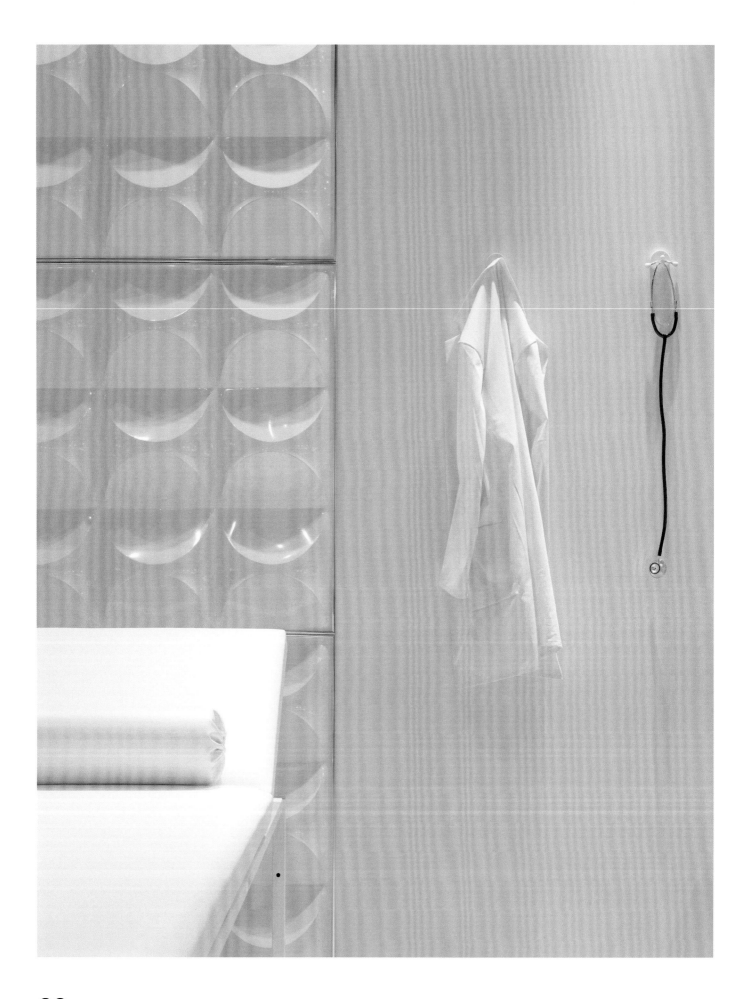

Selected projects

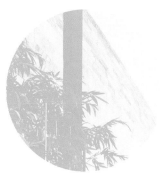

Northwestern Medicine
Central DuPage Hospital

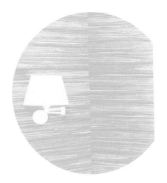

Franziskus
Hospital

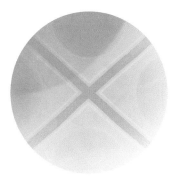

King Juan Carlos
University Hospital

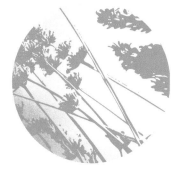

Siloah-Oststadt-
Heidehaus Clinic

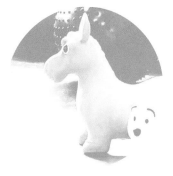

Aiyuhua Hospital
for Women and Children

Patient Room of the
Future Prototype

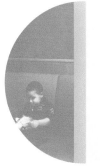

Bayt Abdullah Children's
Hospice (BACCH)

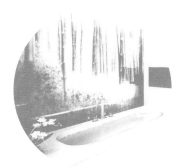

Bumrungrad International
Hospital

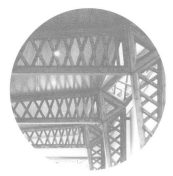

Maggie's
Centres

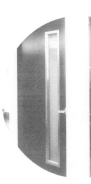

Lenox Hill
Hospital

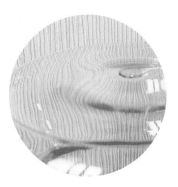

Rems-
Murr Hospital

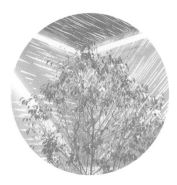

The Salam Centre for
Cardiac Surgery

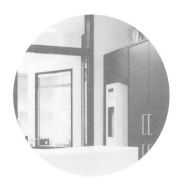

Hospital Engineering Laboratory at the
Fraunhofer-inHaus-Centre

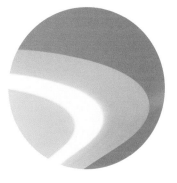

Patient Room 2020
Prototype

Northwestern Medicine Central DuPage Hospital

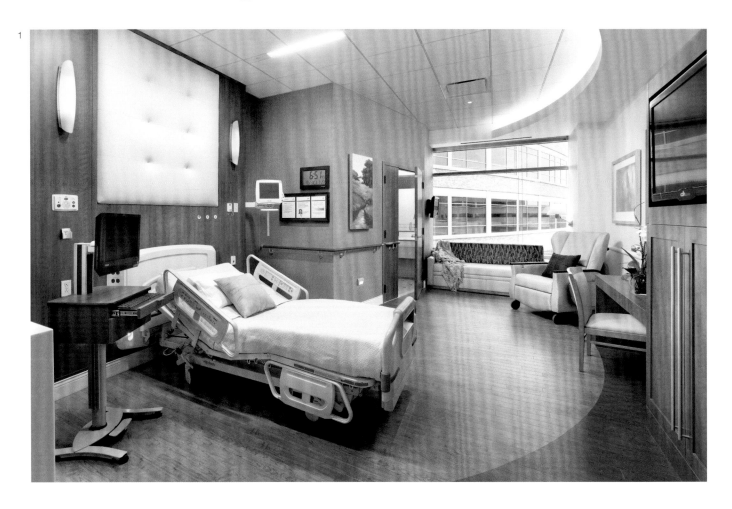

Acute care hospital with
extensive surgical facilities
Winfield, Illinois, USA
Completion: 2011
Design: CallisonRTKL

Northwestern Medicine Central DuPage Hospital was already well known for quality care but wanted to ensure it could continue to attract patient in the future, since patient choice plays an increasingly important role. The hospital took a large-scale renovation of its facilities and a new patient tower as an opportunity to reinvent the patient experience by orienting it around the service, convenience and experience of a five-star hotel.

In addition to mimicking the interior design of a high-end hotel, a study was performed to understand the patient process and flow, nursing patterns and ways to leverage technology in the delivery of care. This was done in order to develop a design for the new bed pavilion that addresses current and future trends in the patient environment and is patient-centric rather than staff- or physician-centric. Consequently, wooden surfaces and accented lighting evoke the atmosphere of a hotel room rather than of a sterile hospital.

The project employs sustainable low-emission materials, improves indoor air quality and incorporates an energy management system to ensure a healthy indoor environment. High-quality surface finishes and a measure of luxury in the choice of light fittings, sanitaryware and other materials add to the sense of comfort. The hospital has been awarded a LEED Silver rating.

1   A patient room with the comfort and atmosphere of a hotel room

2   The lighting reinforces the discreet, high-quality atmosphere of the interior.

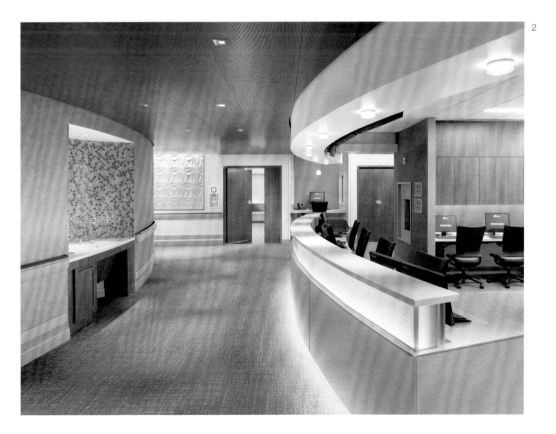

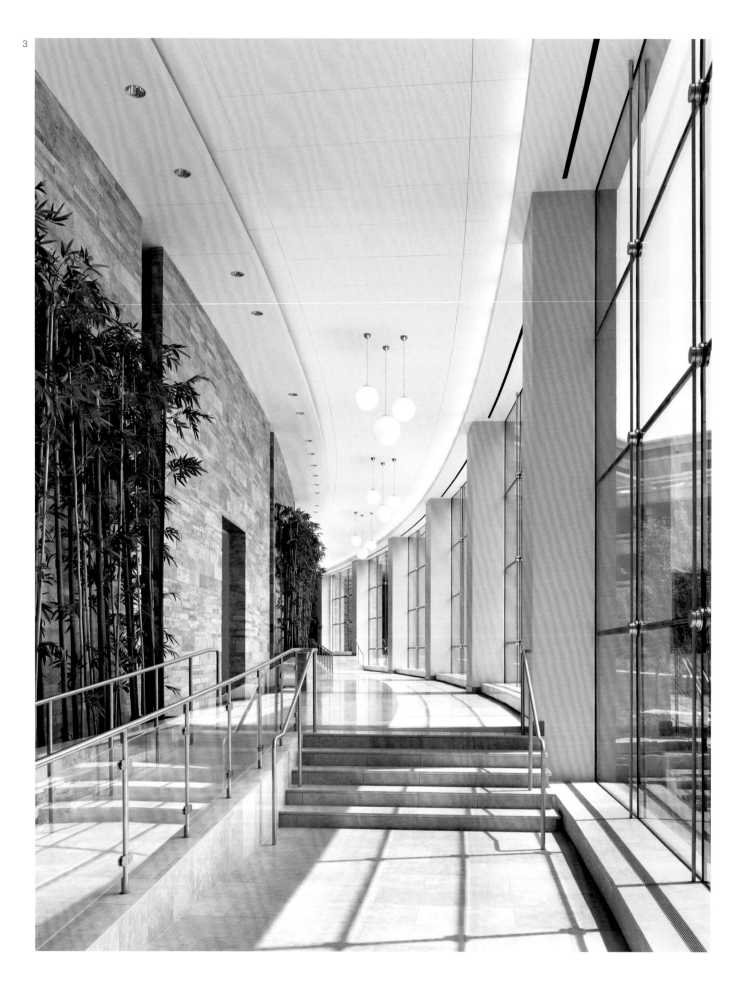

A new pediatric short-stay suite employs bright colours, light and shapes to create a more youthful environment that appeals to young children and teenagers alike. The intention was to create universally appealing interiors that are neither gender- nor age-specific.

The updated Central DuPage Hospital improves patient satisfaction by maximising the patients' sense of security, privacy and comfort.

3   Generous daylight for a sense of well-being

4   The forms of the ceiling recess and floor covering correspond to one another.

5   A circulation space with character rather than linear corridors

6   Corridors with hotel atmosphere – tall, bright spaces with carefully selected fittings

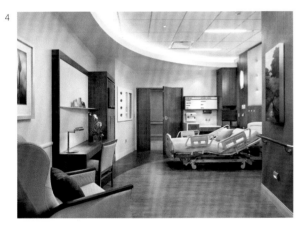

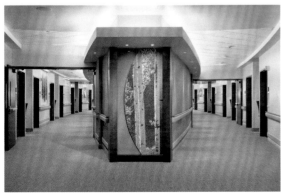

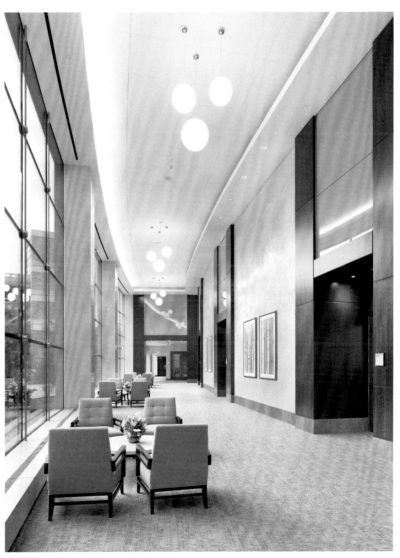

Franziskus Hospital

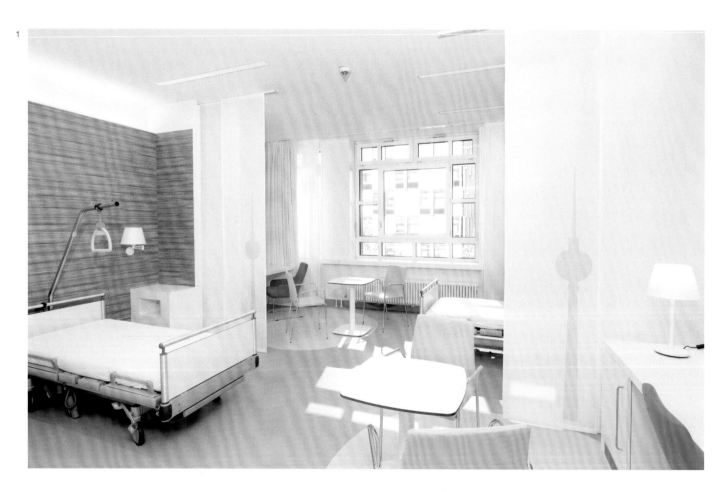

Teaching hospital with
multiple medical specialities
Berlin, Germany
Completion: 2015
Design: Heinle, Wischer
und Partner (HWP)

The Franziskus Hospital in the heart of Berlin is a widely-respected institution run by the Order of Franciscan Sisters. To raise the quality profile of its health-care, the hospital completely renovated two wards in the 1990s extension building, equipping them with premium rooms. The ward has four two-bed rooms and eleven single rooms, along with accompanying lounge areas.

The new patient rooms are equipped with state-of-the-art technology and appointed to a high care standard in the character of a living room, featuring indirect lighting, built-in furniture and high-quality interior and bathroom fittings. Panel curtains and a clever bed arrangement make it possible for two-bed rooms to be divided into separate areas. The various necessary supply lines are incorporated into the built-in fittings so that patients do not have to see them. Graphic elements on the walls depicting stylised silhouettes of Berlin give each room the sense of being of its place.

1   A two-bed room with beds arranged opposite one another

2   Graphic elements mark the entrances to the rooms. Here, part of the iconic "Ampelmänn-chen" walking man figure from East German pedestrian crossing lights.

3   And here, the "Fernsehturm" tower in Berlin.

2

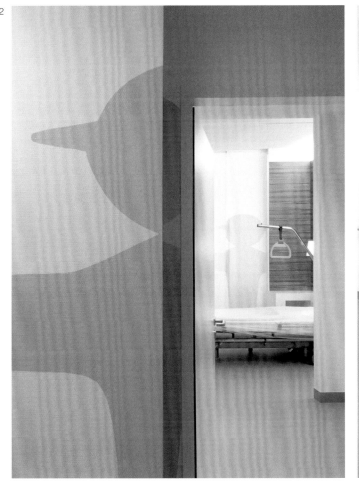

3

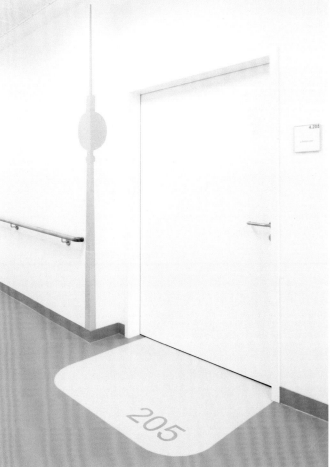

The colour concept – white walls and polished surfaces with bright yellow and green for movable items such as tables and chairs – gives the rooms a bright, refreshing feel. The warm tones of the wood-finish fitted elements create a pleasing contrast. Light-coloured circles within the uniform hygienic linoleum flooring mark certain spots in the rooms in a manner similar to a circular carpet placed on the floor. Corresponding "runners" extend out of the room into the corridor indicating the room number.

4   Wood-effect materials create an
     impression of quality.

5   Floor plan of the ward

6   Bold yellow and green furniture
     add fresh accents to the lounge.

4

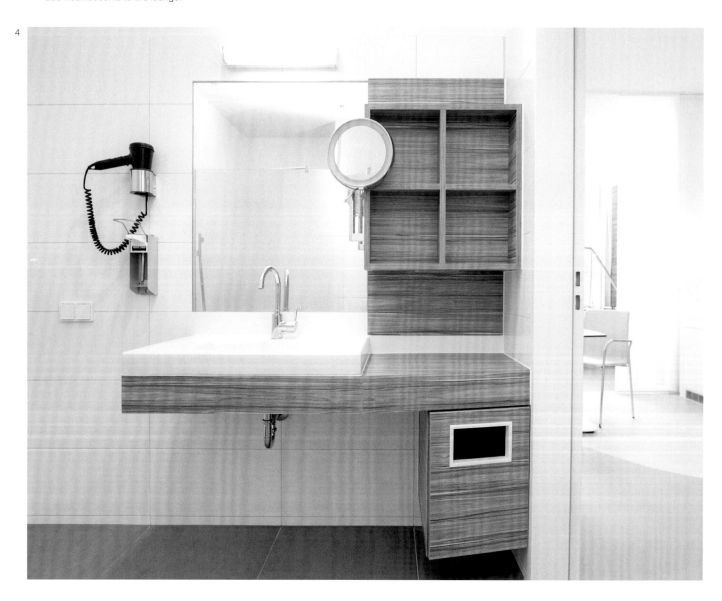

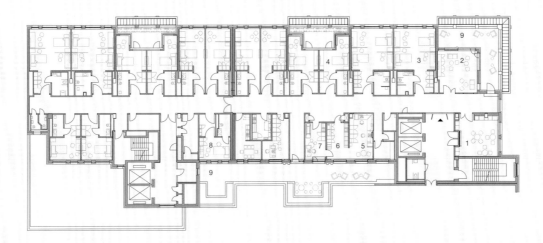

1	Breakfast room	6	Staff room
2	Common room	7	Doctor's examination
3	Two-bed room		room
4	Single-bed room	8	Single-bed isolation room
5	Nursing station	9	Terrace / balcony

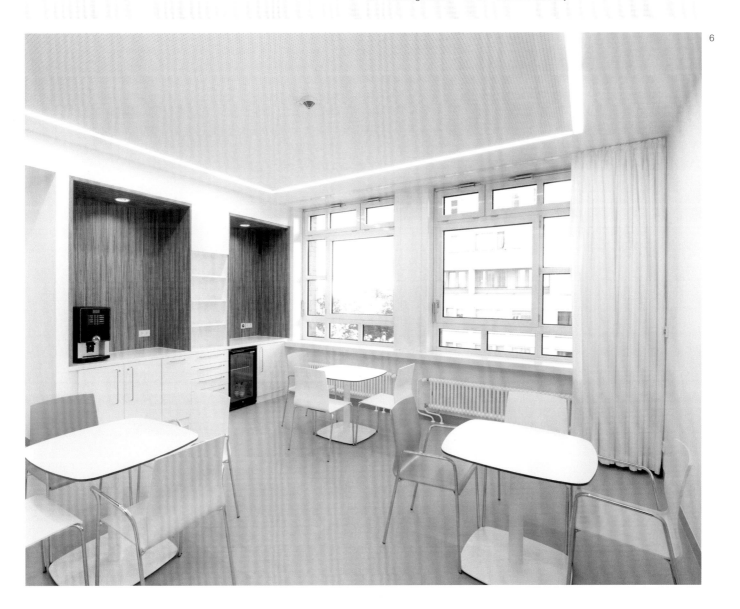

6

King Juan Carlos University Hospital

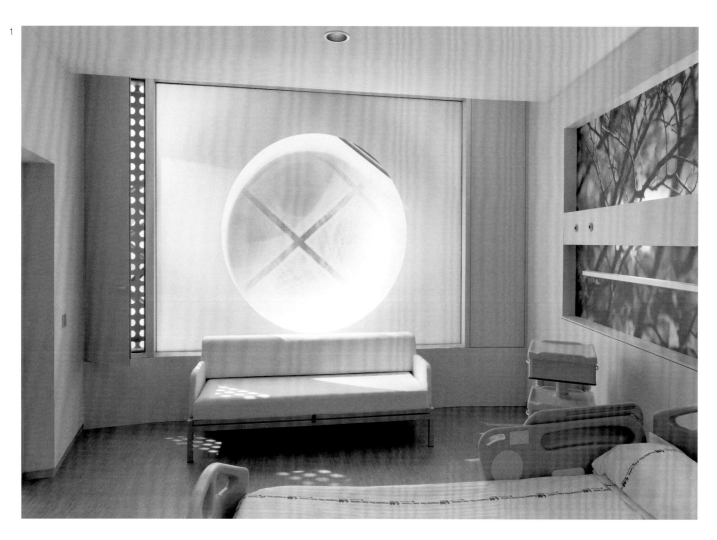

Public hospital
Madrid, Spain
Completion: 2012
Design: Rafael de La-Hoz

While new hospitals must first and foremost provide effective healthcare, their architectural design is often anxiety-inducing, and at times even depressing. The repetition of effective patterns and systems results in monotonous hospital environments. The King Juan Carlos University Hospital recasts the patient as a client with the aim of pairing proven effective healthcare with making the patient the centre of care and attention. The new model combines hospital design with residential design to create an efficient, light and calm interior for rest and recuperation.

Rather than following the model of hotel design, the new design adopts principles from residential design: patients prefer to feel looked after at home rather than tended to in a large hotel-like "curing factory". The interiors feature large images of nature at the head of the bed – the only strong colour in the patient rooms – and are naturally illuminated by circular window openings that afford a view of the world outside. The interior is calm and soothing to reduce patient stress levels.

1   Photographic images of nature are accentuated by indirect lighting.

2   The attractive, circular windows involuntarily attract one's eye.

Two inpatient units are arranged in two separate oval structures that crown the hospital to eliminate long corridors and reduce noise. Each has a concentric, light-filled walkway around the calm interior common atrium. The design addresses the needs of the medical staff and carers and accommodates the desire for each patient to have their own space where they can be "citizens" – i.e. themselves rather than a patient number. It is this approach that contributes to making the patient rooms of the King Juan Carlos University Hospital unique.

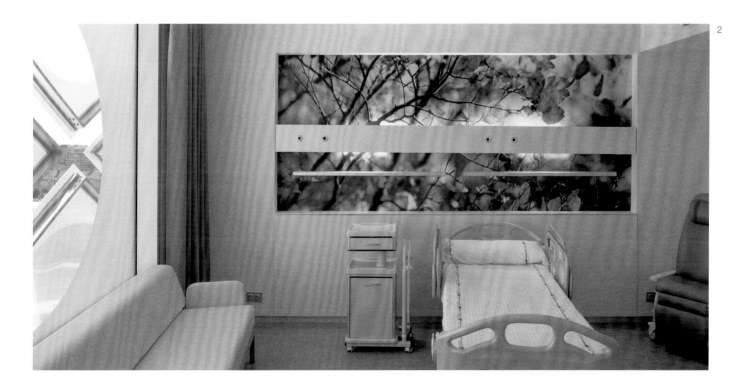
2

Siloah-Oststadt-Heidehaus Clinic

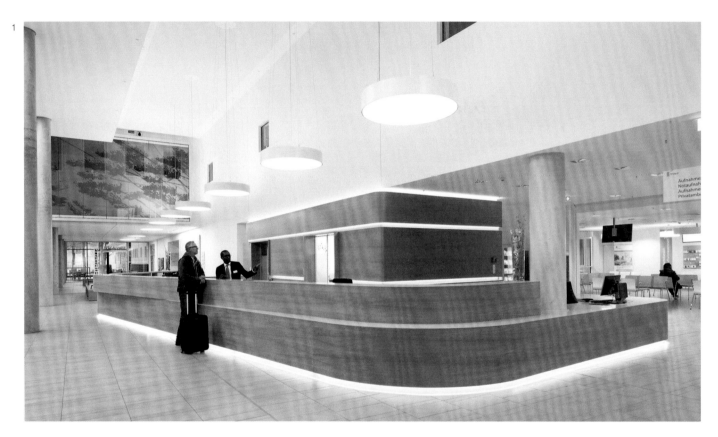

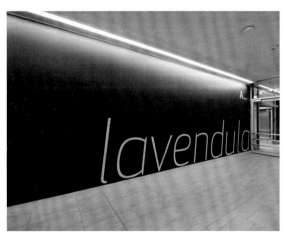

Teaching hospital with multiple medical specialities
Hanover, Germany
Completion: 2014
Design: Sander Hofrichter Architekten (a|sh)

The new "Siloah-Oststadt-Heidehaus Clinic" is a central services hospital (the second-largest class of hospitals in Germany) with a total floor area of 32,000 m² and 535 beds, 40 of which are in a premium services ward.

The interiors are organised around a system of key colours and selected plant motifs that denote the respective wards. The colour green picks up the colour of the planting in the adjoining internal courtyards. Stylised large-format graphics of the leaves and blossoms of the plants in the courtyards grace the walls of each wing. The rooms around the "Gingko Courtyard", for example, feature not only Gingko motifs on the walls but also selected verses of poems by Goethe.

Strong shades of red, yellow and violet serve as atmospheric references to a corresponding medicinal plant – hibiscus, calendula and lavender – and as wayfinding indicators denoting each of the three patient room wings. Each of these key colours defines the interiors of the nursing wards in the respective wing from the main corridor to the lift to the patient rooms. Out of the windows, one can see the respective plant growing on the roof below. Details of the blossom recur on the walls as graphical motifs, paired with verses of poetry and background information on the medicinal plants. The interior design corresponds to its respective natural surroundings, connecting the two and creating a harmonious whole.

1   A large reception block welcomes visitors and patients as they arrive.

2   Deep violet is the key colour of the lavender area.

3   Graphic representations of lavender as decorative accents in the patient room

3

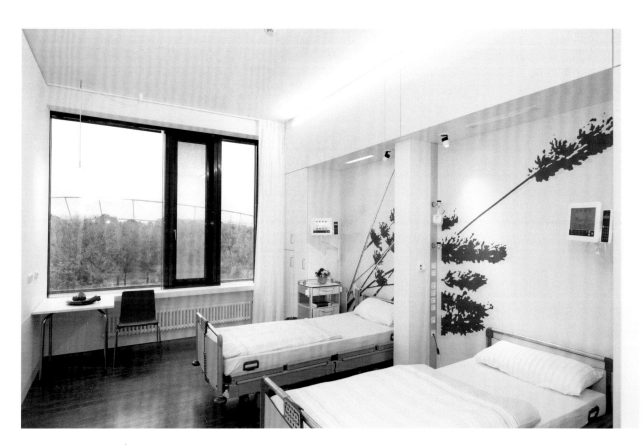

4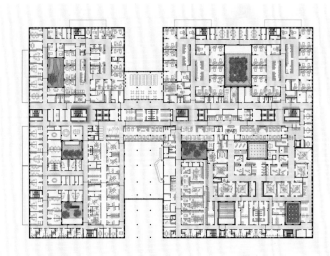

5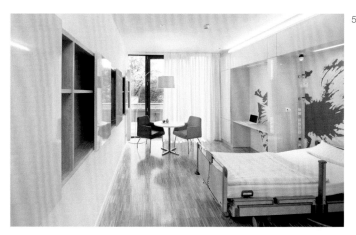

6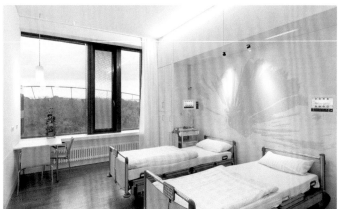

7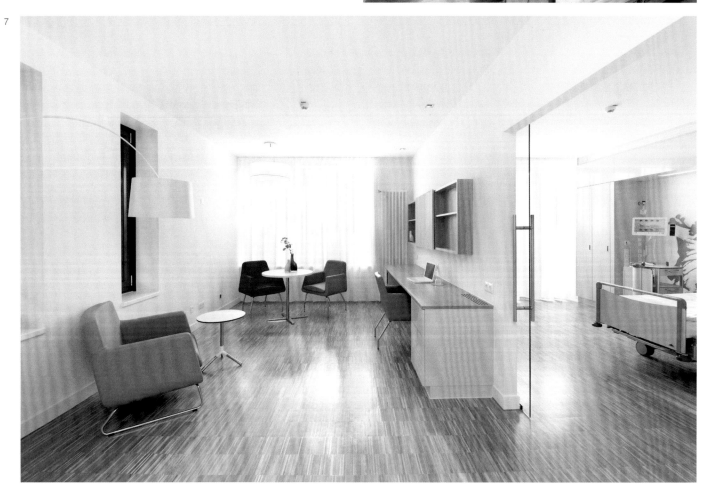

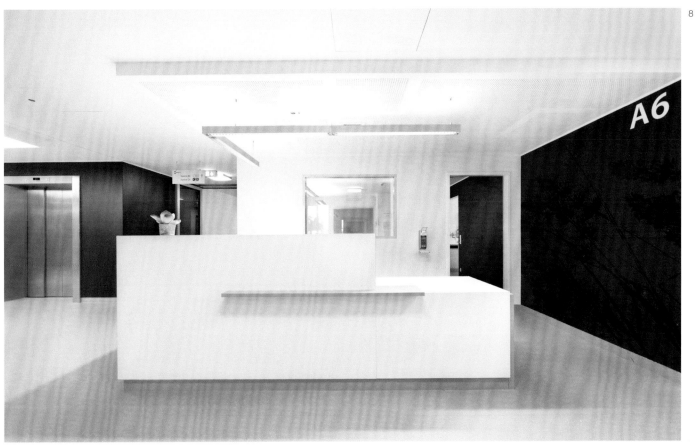

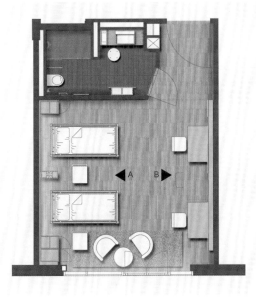

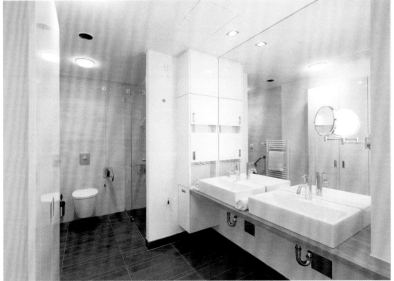

4   Floor plan

5   A single premium room

6   Two-bed room with calendula wall graphic

7   A living area with armchair, desk and sitting area in a premium suite

8   The nursing station in the lavender wing

9   Floor plan of a premium two bed room with enough space for two desks

10 Bathroom interior with twin washbasin in a premium room

Aiyuhua Hospital for Women and Children

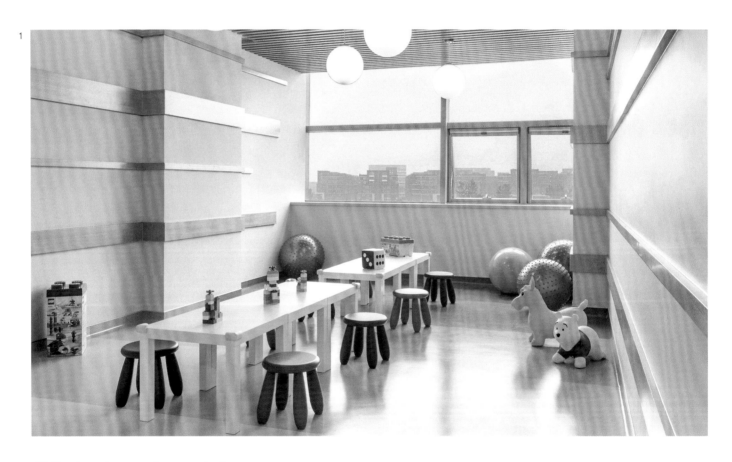

Clinic for obstetrics
and gynaecology
Beijing, China
Completion: 2014
Design: HKS architects

Aiyuhua Hospital for Women and Children is China's first women's and children's medical centre. The hospital provides world-class prenatal care, obstetrics, maternity monthly stay service, paediatrics and child health management services.

As demand for women's and children's health services expands, providers must raise the bar for the patient care they provide. Hospital staff need to provide care not just for the patients but also for their families to ensure the overall well-being of the patients. The design goals for the hospital were therefore to create a family-centred as well as staff-focussed healing environment with spacious patient rooms, waiting areas and play rooms. Spaces are designed to be human and approachable without compromising on high-tech digital equipment or on sustainability. The rooms are painted in pleasant blue, green and yellow pastel colours that are typical for the region. Elegant lounges, wood finishes and light accents are combined with bright, child-friendly colour schemes.

1   Colourful pastel colours define
    the playroom.

2   Child-oriented graphic elements
    and colours

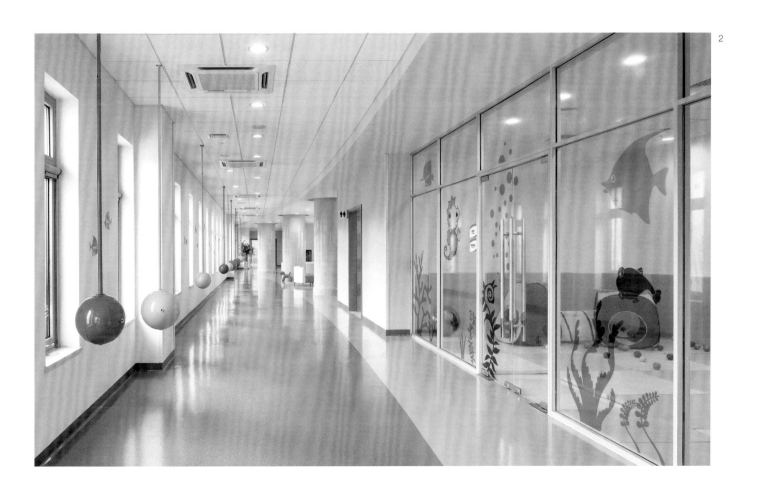

2

The hospital's design makes maximum use of natural light and spacious interiors to create a calm healing environment for women and children alike. Light and colour are used for wayfinding to define destinations and indicate pathways, providing intuitive navigational cues to assist patient and visitor orientation. This scheme can be expanded horizontally or vertically using further colours and shades to accommodate future additions to the hospital.

3   A comfortable
    single-bed room

4   A pleasant, comfortable
    waiting area

5   The canopy over the
    bed creates a sense of
    shelter.

3

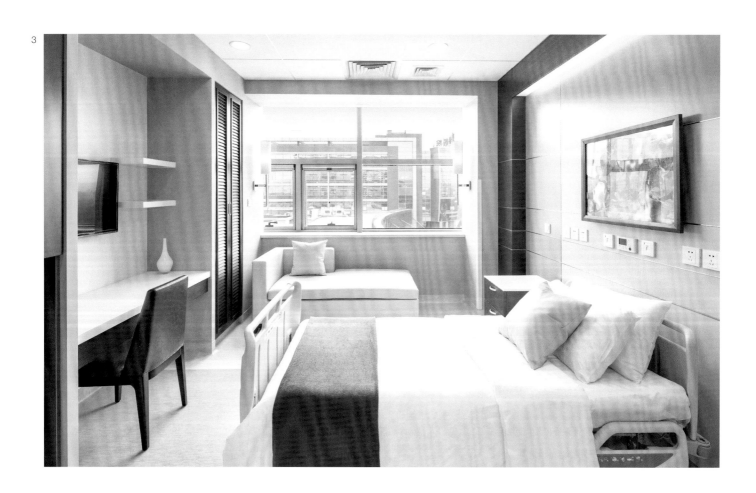

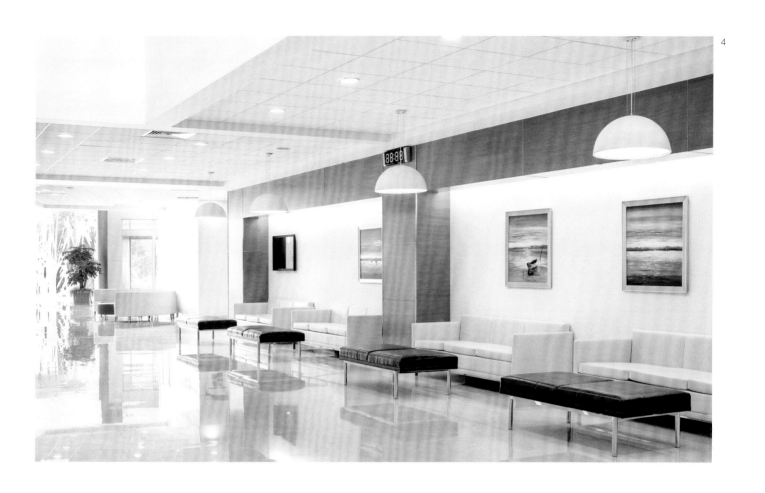

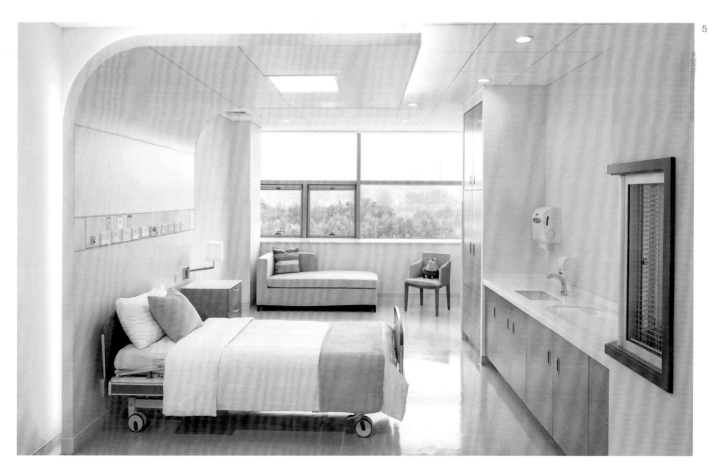

Patient Room of the Future Prototype

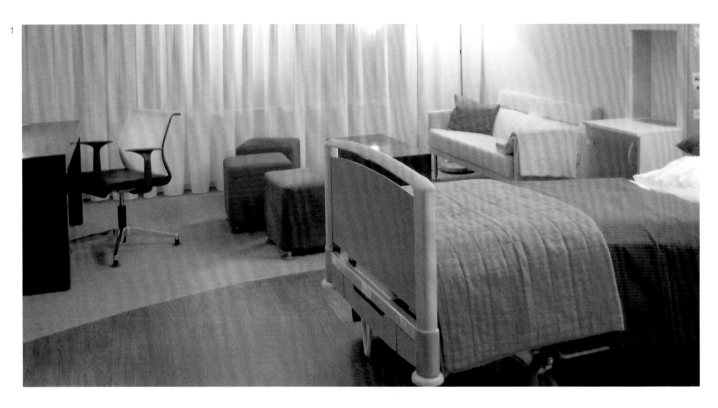

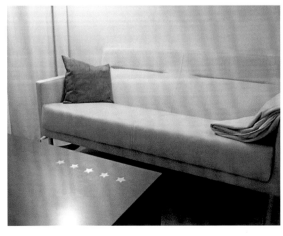

Mock-up patient room for
Forum MAD succidia
Verlag / medical lounge
Berlin, Germany
Completion: 2006
Design: 100% interior,
Sylvia Leydecker

The design for the Patient Room of the Future was realised as a full-scale mock-up in 2006 as part of a conference in Berlin's medical lounge, and at the time represented a milestone in the design of patient rooms. Two key parameters inform the design of the single room: the desire to create a more hotel-like character and the intention to incorporate smart materials. Hygiene was a central focus, achieved, for example, by avoiding hard-to-clean gaps and the use of hygienic materials and surfaces.

The patient room for private healthcare patients has a comfortable, homely atmosphere designed to create a feeling of well-being and security. The palette of materials and colours – cherry wood with contrasting wenge wood, along with warm orange and cream tones – has been specially devised to communicate a high-quality atmosphere. A graphic motif on the ceiling enlivens the space and incorporates the ceiling as part of the room design.

The Patient Room of the Future does away with the utilitarian wet cell of traditional patient rooms and replaces it with a larger-than-normal, attractively designed space that can justifiably be called a bathroom. Bold accents, such as the canary-yellow washbasin, made of a hygienic composite mineral, provide an added element of surprise. A sliding door ensures peace and privacy and the curved dividing wall subtly guides one's passage on both sides of the wall.

Not visible but practical is the use of additional high-tech nanotechnology-enhanced materials such as anti-bacterial varnishes and light switches, air-cleansing wall paints and curtains, hydrophobic and vapour-permeable wall coverings instead of wall tiles, self-cleaning floor tiles and easy-to-clean surfaces in the bathroom.

1   The colour and material concept communicates a sense of warmth and shelter and conveys the comfort and atmosphere of a hotel room.

2   A sofa offers a possibility for patients to move closer and offer one another support.

3   A bathroom that is quite different to the typical tiled wet cell.

4   Graphic elements on the ceiling let one's eyes wander.

5   The mock-up from outside

3
4
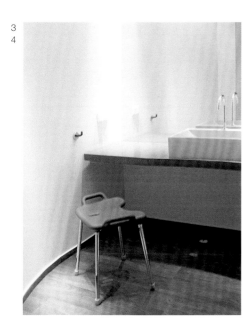
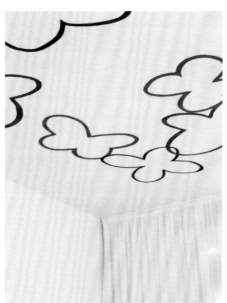
5
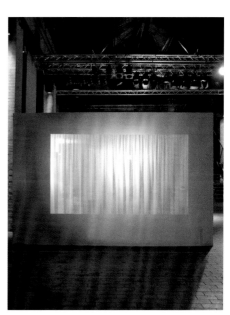

Bayt Abdullah Children's Hospice (BACCH)

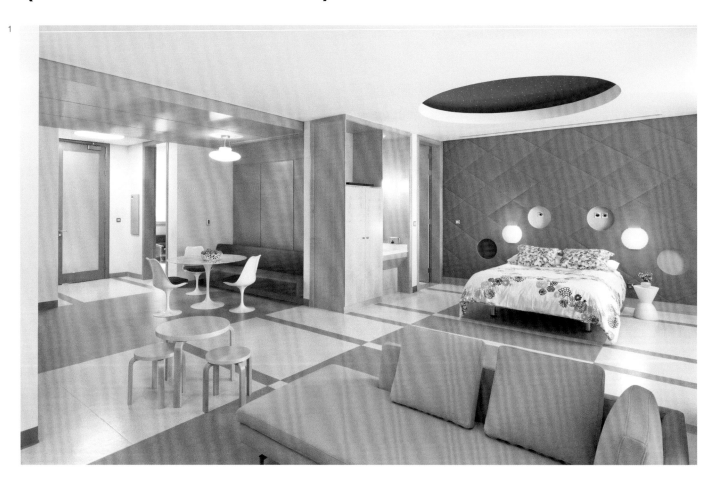

1

Paediatric palliative care hospice
Sulaibikhat, Kuwait
Completion: 2012
Design: NBBJ Architectural
and Specialist Interior Designers;
Architecture: Alia Al Ghunaim

The Bayt Abdullah Children's Hospice (BACCH) is the only palliative care centre in the Middle East and one of the largest in the world. BACCH aims to give the care they need and psychosocial support for children with advanced cancer and their families in their spiritual journey as they navigate the difficulties of dealing with this life-limiting illness.

Life for these children can be chaotic and scary, so the design objective was to give them control of their environment and to enable them to live as normal a life as possible. A variety of places for playing, including an art room, library or video game area is available.

1 Strong colours and deep orange lend the room a positive atmosphere.

2 Seating areas for different needs – from open communication to places for sheltered conversation

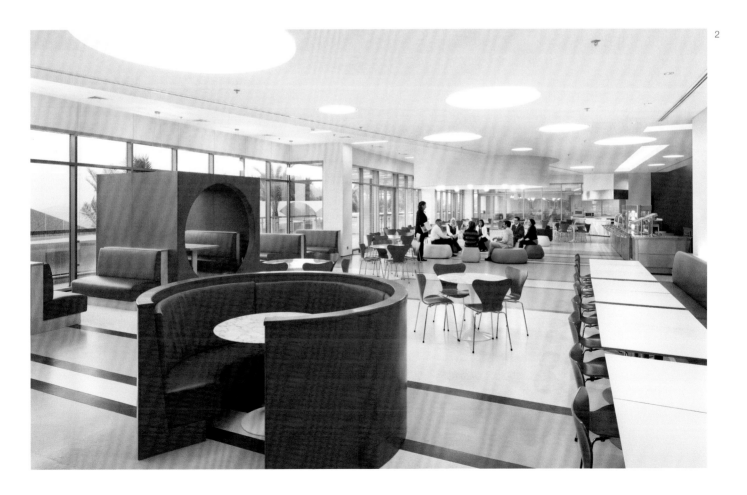

2

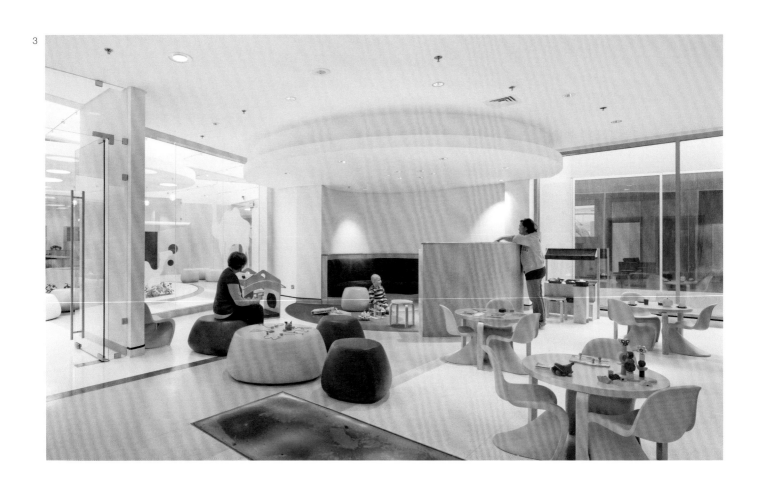

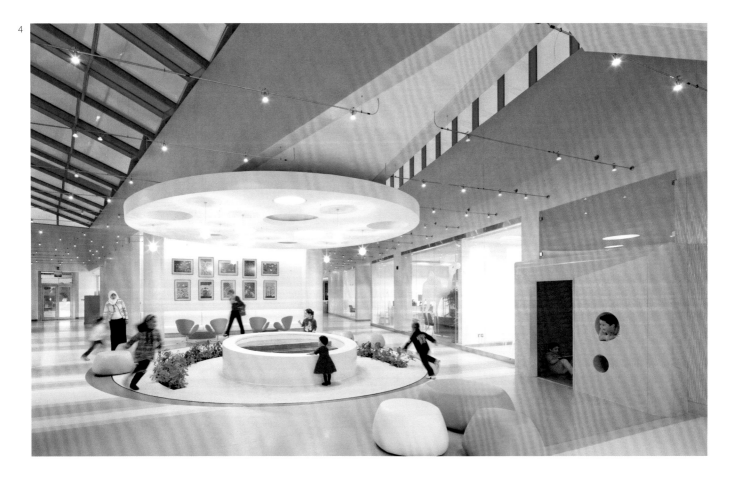

Families can select a level of privacy appropriate to their needs by choosing an inpatient suite or one of eleven private chalets. Inside the chalets, a tone-in-tone colour scheme conveys a sense of serenity, with warm colours and lighting to create a residential ambience.

The inpatient suites are designed to resemble a home setting rather than a traditional hospital room, with an atmosphere conducive to regular family life, play and staying overnight. The design supports families in all stages on the journey of their child's illness, differentiating for instance between the needs of first-time patients and repeat visitors. Child-centric design is evident throughout Bayt Abdullah. Light accents bring out the colours, and bright and bold red, blue, yellow and green colours dominate the interiors. Graphics with typical regional motifs, such as camels, contribute to creating a fun, playful atmosphere to reduce anxiety at a very stressful time.

3   Sufficient space to play and enjoy is integral to the concept.

4   Areas that stimulate imagination distract from the illness.

5   Graphic elements, such as the camel, create a connection with the region.

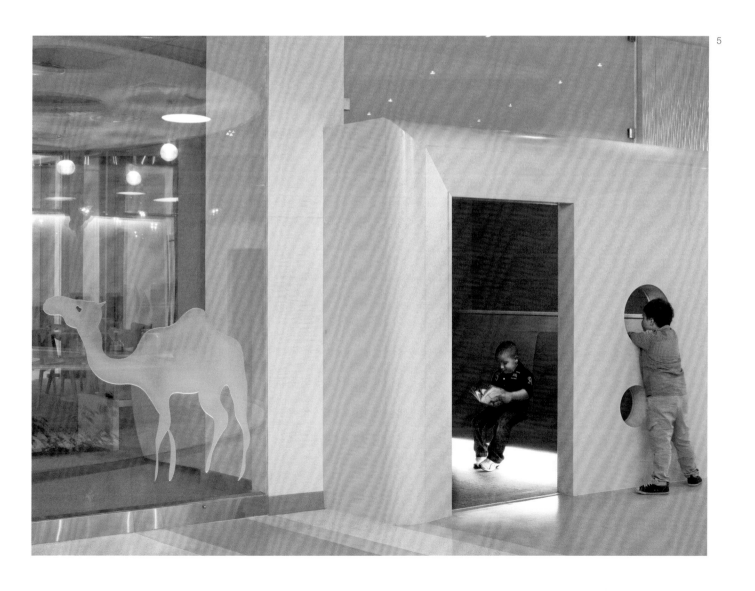

5

Bumrungrad International Hospital

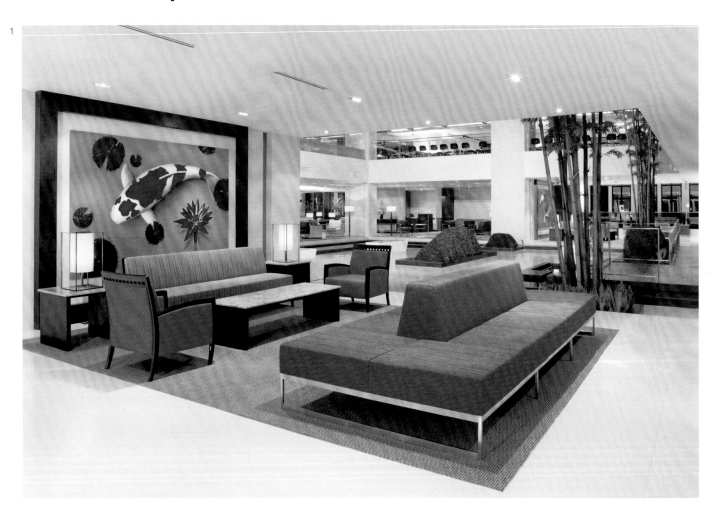

Multiple-speciality hospital
Bangkok, Thailand
Completion: 2008
Design: dwp

As part of the renovation and upgrading of its facilities, the renowned Bumrungrad International Hospital introduced a new calm, contemporary atmospheric interior design that is welcoming for patients and visitors alike. Using natural materials, tonal colour palettes, accent lighting solutions, and custom signage systems and graphics, the new interiors are designed to evoke a sense of comfort, wellness and warmth with an underlying "Zen" theme in all the spaces.

Building on the success of this recent renovation, a similar approach has been adopted for the interior design of their labour and delivery ward. The inspiration for the design comes from the purity of newborn babies and the healing power of nature, with the intention of creating a light and soothing ambience. Natural colours and materials, artwork and other elements have been combined with careful detailing and attention to detail, and medical equipment has been integrated smartly to create an integral wellness and medical experience right up until after the delivery of the baby.

A palette of wood-clad walls, brown hues and red accents has been used to create a warm atmosphere. The lighting concept employs a mixture of direct and indirect light, highlighting walls, contours and ceilings to create an atmosphere more akin to that of a hotel than a hospital. Soft and light shades of colour in the patients' bathrooms along with wall-height images of nature enhance the sense of well-being to recover easily.

1   The refined atmosphere of a first-class hotel helps create a sense of trust.

2   A bright, clear and clean bathroom interior

2

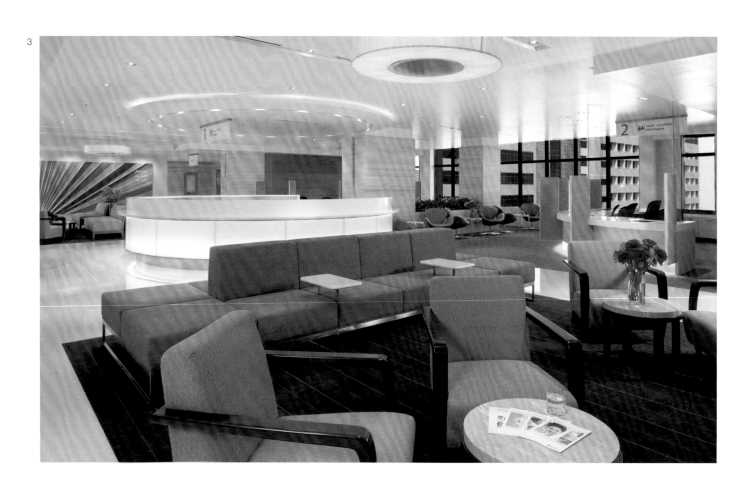

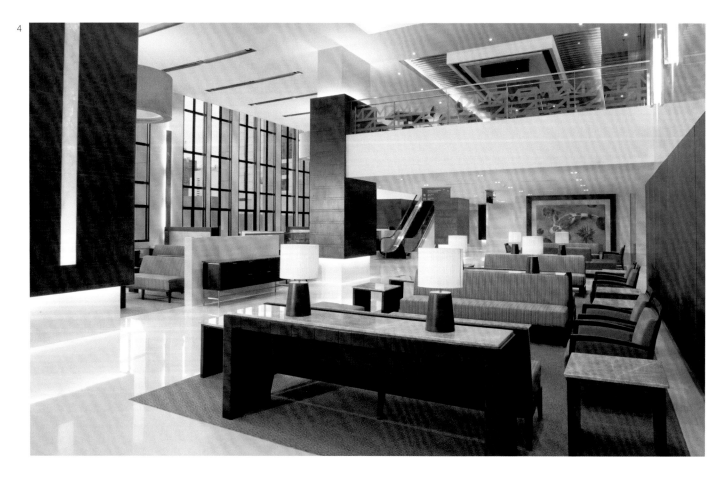

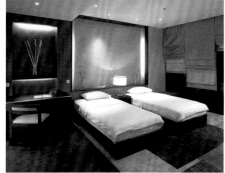

5

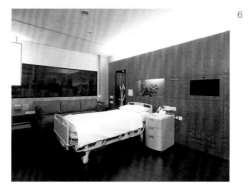

6

3　An atmospheric reception area flanked by a comfortable waiting zone

4　Pleasant, subdued lighting in the waiting area

5　A two-bed room allows a relative to stay.

6　Muted colours in a single-bed room create a sense of class and comfort.

7　Floor plan

8　Elegant, high-quality interiors

9　The nurses' station in operation

7

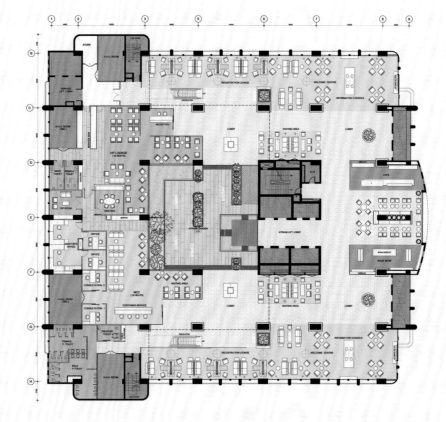

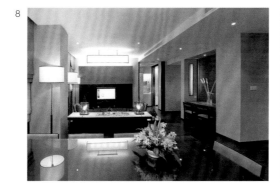

8

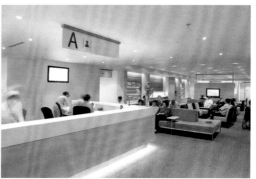

9

Maggie's Centres

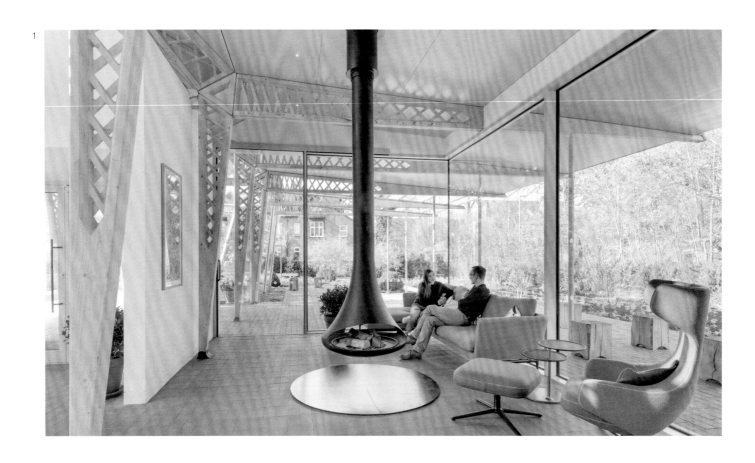

Drop-in support centres for people
with cancer and their relatives
United Kingdom
Completion: 1996–2016
Design: various. Shown here are centres by
CZWG, Foster + Partners, Kisho Kurokawa
architect & associates and Garbers & James,
Richard Murphy Architects

The various Maggie's Centres in Great Britain are examples of "humane havens" – healthcare buildings with a human spirit. Named after and founded by Maggie Keswick Jencks, the wife of architectural theorist and landscape architect Charles Jencks, the centres are dedicated to providing support for people with cancer. The success of the model in England has led to the establishment of further centres outside Europe, for example in Hong Kong and Tokyo. The centres provide free practical, emotional and social support to cancer patients and their families without the need for prior formal registration.

The buildings are not only central to the Maggie's concept, but also to how they operate as open, friendly, informal and people-focussed environments. Luxury is less important than the outlook of the centres and their work. Numerous well-known architects have designed Maggie's Centres, including Richard Rogers, Zaha Hadid and Norman Foster.

Maggie's Centres are designed around the needs of people with cancer. Their aim is to counteract isolation by providing a place for human contact and friendship to show them they are not alone. The rooms of the centre embody this idea by providing an easy, relaxed atmosphere for informal interaction. Deliberately devoid of any anxiety-inducing institutional character, they are pleasant, humane and inviting places that place no expectations on their visitors. As independent centres, free of the stipulations of clients, their design communicates a sense of community and togetherness rather than the institutional character of a medical facility. Each centre has direct contact to nature, and the building designs delight in making the most of light, form and good-quality materials – without being dogmatic or severe – to create uplifting environments for living with cancer in a protective and supportive atmosphere.

2

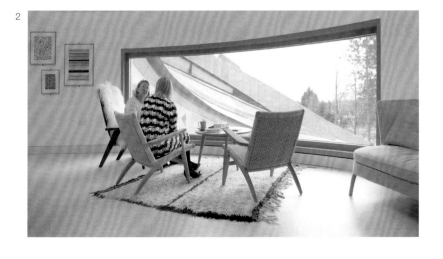

1   Comfortable places to sit, talk and relax are part of the concept. Foster + Partners, Maggie's Centre, Manchester, England

2   Comfortable chairs, a carpet, a couple of pictures on the wall and a view outside create the perfect environment for a good conversation. Kisho Kurokawa architect & associates and Garbers & James, Maggie's Centre, Swansea, Wales

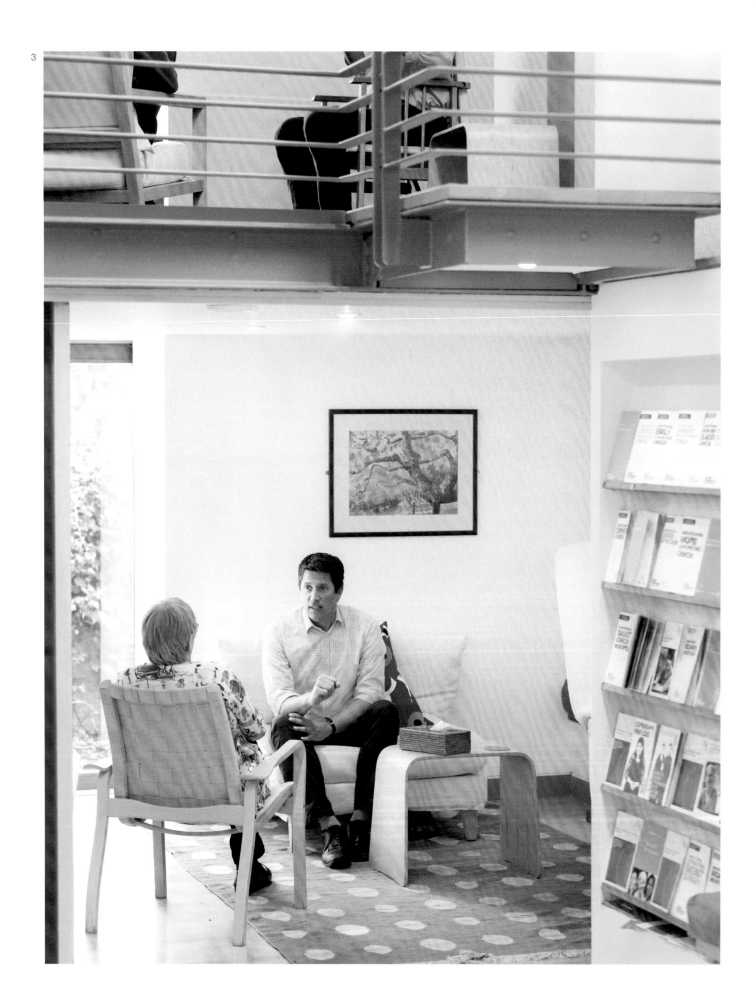

3 Places to talk in a human environment are essential. Richard Murphy Architects, Maggie's Centre, Edinburgh, Scotland

4 A homely atmosphere creates a sense of "normality". CZGW Architects, Maggie's Centre, Nottingham, England

5 Perfect living room atmosphere with potted plants and delicate wood supports. Foster + Partners, Maggie's Centre, Manchester, England

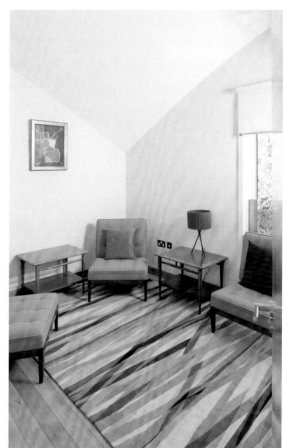

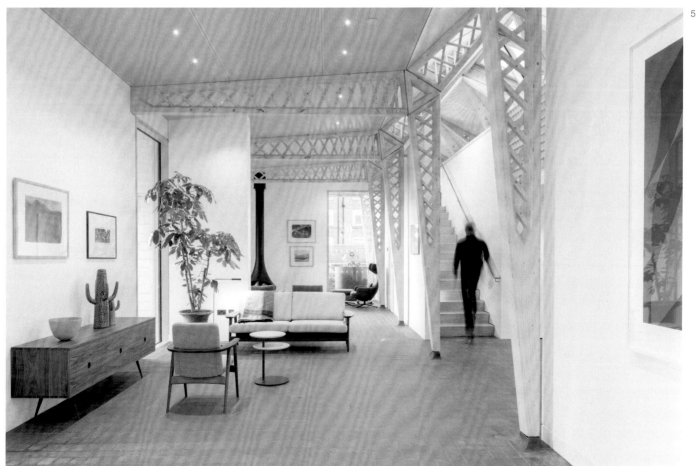

Lenox Hill Hospital

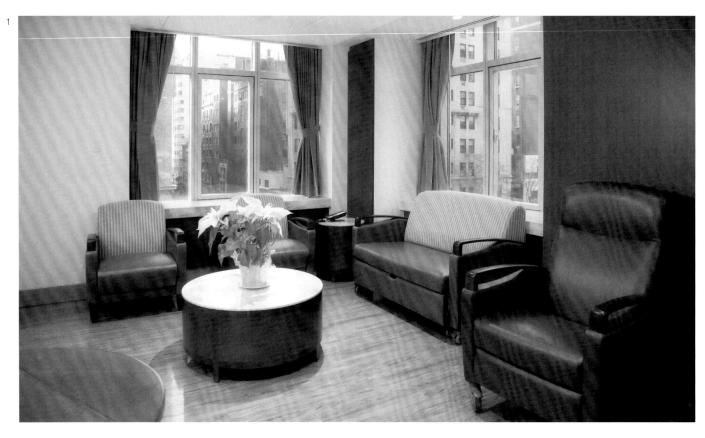

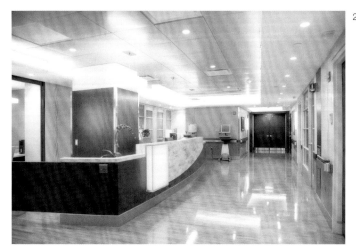

Acute care hospital
with multiple medical
specialities
New York, USA
Completion: 2013
Design: e4h Architecture

This extremely fast-track project, including an approx. 60 m² state-of-the-art operating room coupled with an approx. 470 m² luxury inpatient suite, was designed for a leading prostate surgeon in New York, USA. The inpatient unit can accommodate ten patients with all amenities in a hotel-like environment.

Although LEED certification was not applied for due to the tight construction schedule, sustainability was a major concern in its design and the choice of materials. The design makes connections with the outside world and nearby Central Park, reinforcing these with images of nature – a large wall-height print of cherry blossoms in the reception, for example – to focus attention away from the medical procedure. The principles of patient empowerment and family support underline the concept of the facility.

Dark cherrywood panelling and light grey and beige surfaces create a soothing, warm interior of contrasting materials. Large, dark-brown armchairs, typical of American interiors, invite patients and guests to relax. All finishes are selected and detailed to minimise hard-to-clean areas, helping to prevent the spread of infection and contamination. In the bedrooms, medical supply lines are hidden from view and floor finishes are chosen to reduce the risk of slips and falls. Sound transmission is mitigated by acoustic design and the selection of materials with high noise reduction coefficients.

The combination of these Evidence-Based Design elements allow the institution to focus on the outstanding provision of care and on improving patient outcomes.

1   Heavy armchairs create a focus in the room.

2   Wood in combination with varied lighting creates a sense of class and comfort.

3   Wood panelling creates a homely character.

4   Images of cherry blossoms as a decorative accent

3
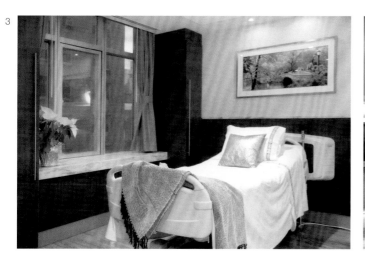

4
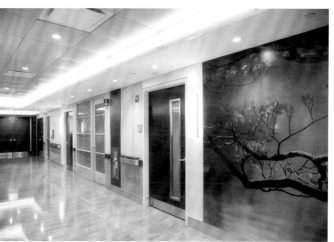

Rems-Murr Hospital

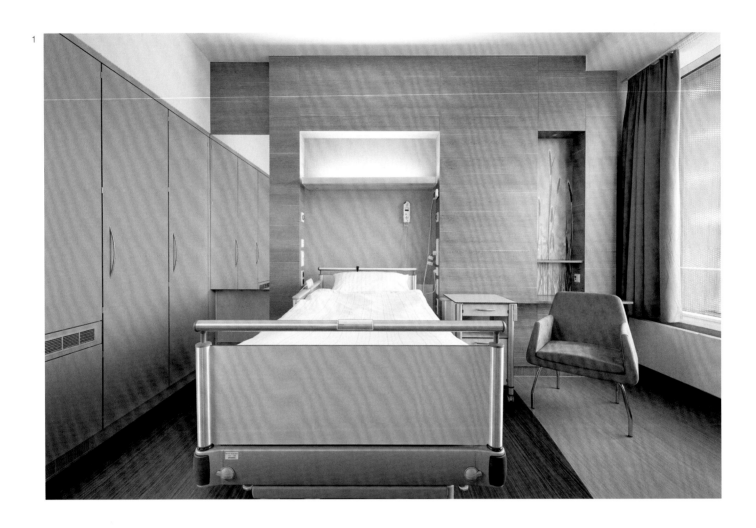

Hospital with multiple
medical specialities
Winnenden, Germany
Completion: 2014
Design: 100% interior,
Sylvia Leydecker

1 Muted colours and subtle natural tones have been used to create a comfortable healing environment with a hotel-like atmosphere.

2 A high-quality, discreetly lettered door opens onto a patient room.

3 Green colour accents – a wall niche with a photographic detail of grasses behind hygienic glass and a comfortable armchair with textured upholstery

The new Rems-Murr Hospital includes both entire premium wards and individual premium rooms in other wards that fulfil private health insurance criteria for comfort and a corresponding hotel-room atmosphere in all respects.

Evidence-Based Design has been used to create a healing environment that embodies the clinic's medical care philosophy and provides optimal conditions for patients to recover. The design language draws inspiration from nature and the image of long grasses swaying in the wind. Different sand and earth tones continue the natural theme, contrasting pleasingly with fresh green accents to create a harmonious balance.

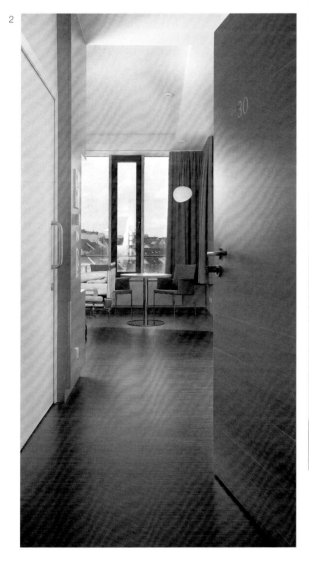

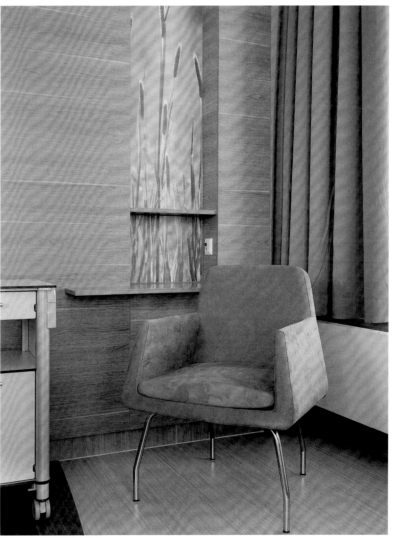

The design of the clinic's maternity ward, on the other hand, appeals specifically to the tastes of the predominantly younger clientele. All hygienic requirements are fulfilled down to the last detail with clearly delineated, easy-to-clean, hygienic surface materials. A variable lighting concept creates a warm atmosphere, even on grey days. Images of nature and discreet surface textures make subtle reference to nature, while points of colour in the (non-brown) maternity room wallpaper lend the room a youthful, joyful atmosphere.

The technical equipment – which patients often find disconcerting – is hidden behind a vertical panel at the head of the bed. Generous views of the surrounding landscape round off the pleasant atmosphere of the room, but patients can also darken the room by closing the curtains as required.

4   A healing environment through and through. The image of grasses also recurs in the premium room's bathroom.

5–6   Sketches of the patient room interior

7   Warm colours evoke vitality.

8   Transparent plastic contrasts with the vertical grass-like texture of the wall covering.

9   Calm, clear interiors with a view into a room

10   The maternity ward room for private healthcare patients addresses the needs of the mother, child and visitors.

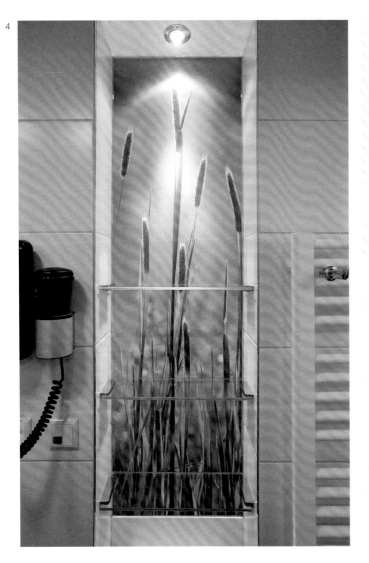

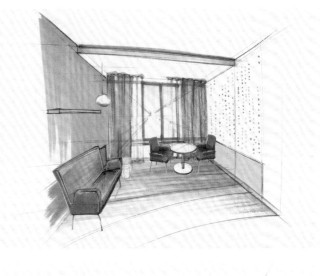

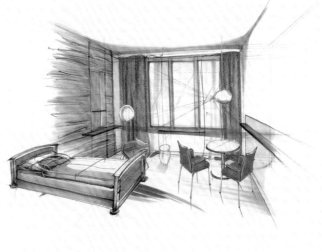

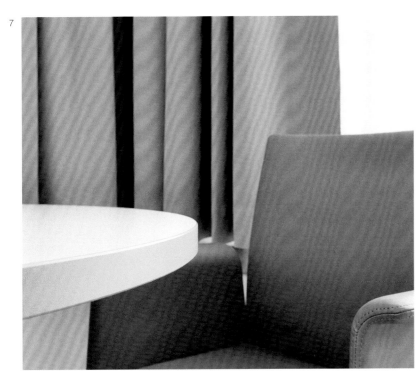

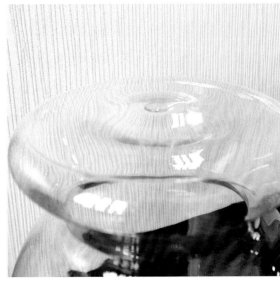

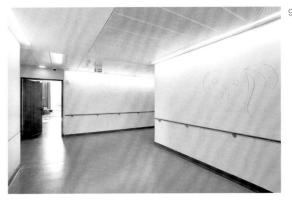

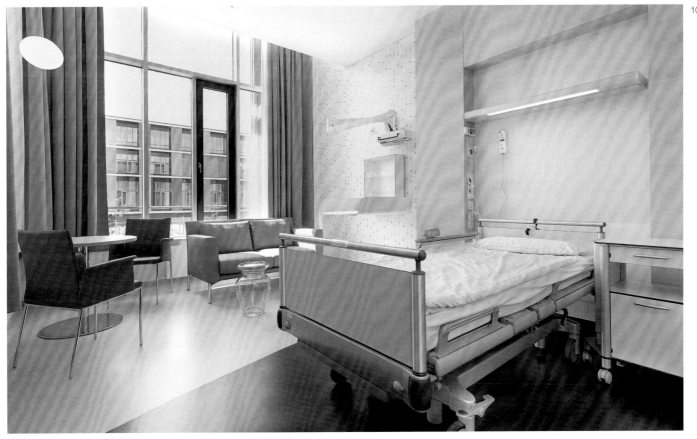

The Salam Centre for Cardiac Surgery

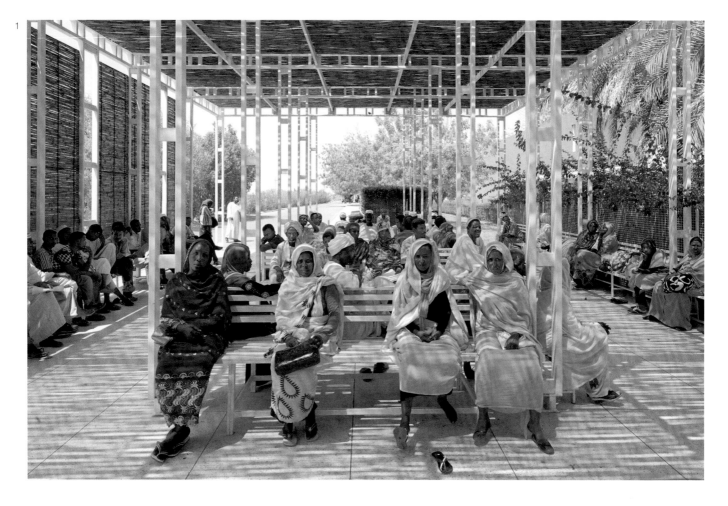

Centre for cardiac surgery
for adults and children
Khartoum, Sudan
Completion: 2007
Design: TAMassociati

The Salam Centre for Cardiac Surgery was awarded the prestigious Aga Khan Award for Architecture in 2013. Run by the Italian humanitarian organisation and NGO "Emergency", it delivers a responsible, efficient and inspiring model of health services.

The hospital on the banks of Blue Nile has 63 beds and is situated in a garden complex where it encloses a courtyard. This direct link to its natural surroundings creates a clear, approachable environment to facilitate healing and recuperation. The hospital's aim is to provide the fundamental right of health to everyone and its design followed a bottom-up process involving local, political and social stakeholders that took into account the specific local topographical and aesthetic qualities without sacrificing the overarching vision for excellent medical care.

1   The air-permeable roof of woven plant stems provides shade without obstructing a pleasant breeze.

2   The bright, white pavilion is open to members of all religions for prayer and meditation and reflects the sunlight.

3   Trees as a natural element within the pavilion

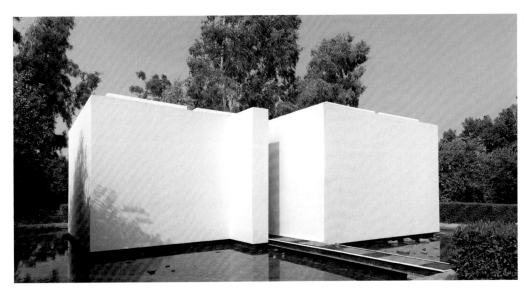

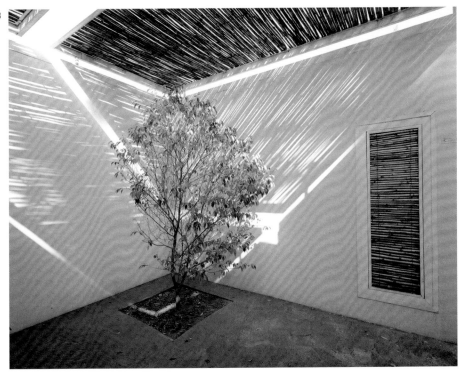

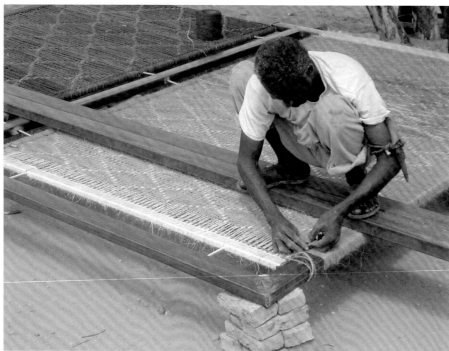

4

5

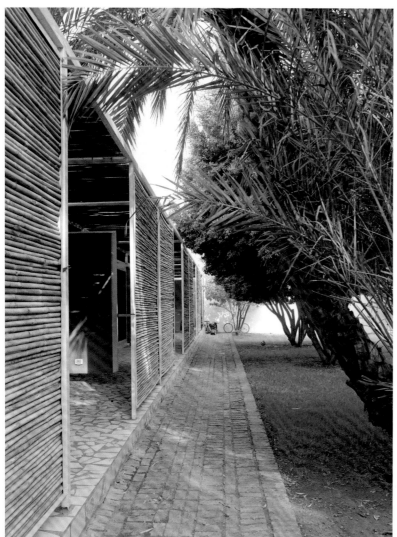

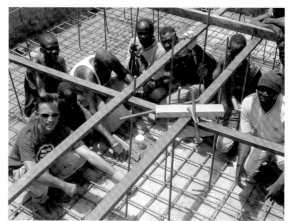

6

4   Local production of woven mats made of plant fibres

5   Nature is everywhere.

6   Teamwork

7   Light and shadow create a cool place to sit and wait in the sub-Saharan climate.

8   Waiting patiently in the corridor

9   The combination of blue and white creates a cool impression, reducing the subjective perception of the air temperature.

The hospital uses economical and accessible materials and employs mixed ventilation modes to address the local climate, which can reach temperatures in excess of 40-50°C and is frequently dusty due to the "Haboub" desert winds. The interiors are naturally illuminated with shade provided by woven screens and natural planting, and materials and details have been selected and designed to reduce the sense of hospitalisation. The less clinical the surroundings, the better the patients will feel and the stronger the focus on the values of caring and preserving life.

The state-of-the-art hospital has had a tremendous impact. Its example and vision have encouraged the establishment of further medical centres of excellence in other African countries.

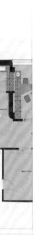

1   Two-bed room as th
     model with numerou
     invisible sensors.

2   The nursing station

3   Floor plan of the wa

4   Bathroom with disa
     fittings and floor-lev
     tray

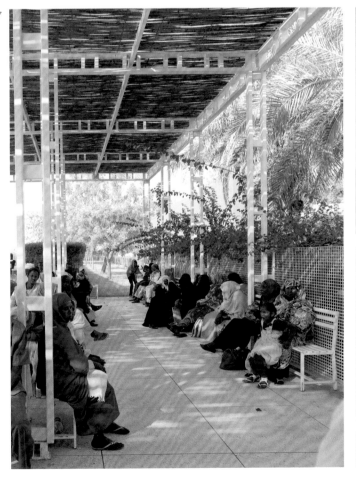

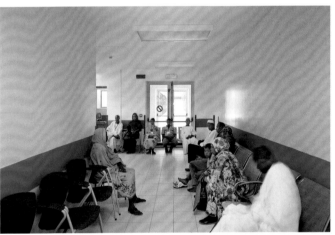

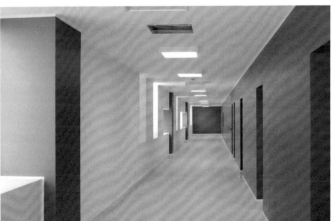

141

Ho
La

at the

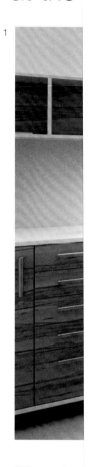

Testin
as a re
collab
Duisbu
Projec
Devel
Institu
Thöne

142

Patient Room 2020
Prototype

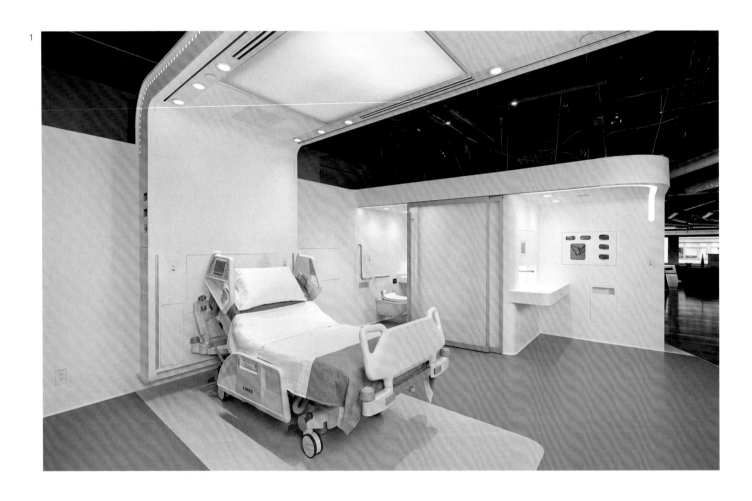

Next-generation inpatient
care prototype
New York, USA
Completion: 2013
Design: NXT Health in
collaboration with Evans &
Paul and Dolan & Traynor

144

This prototype of a future, next-generation patient room is the product of a collaboration between industry partners and opened to the public in New York City, USA, at the design studio of its main sponsor DuPont Corian. The predominant material is solid surface, which is very suitable for healthcare environments due to its hygienic characteristics. While patient rooms and healing environments typically favour natural colours over the perceived sterility of white interiors, here the white colour of the material and its soft contours, clean lines and matt finish, heighten the impression of hygiene. More than 35 product and service partners contributed to the design of the Patient Room 2020.

The approx. 40 m² prototype is technology-driven, leveraging an extensive range of technologies for the five key parts of the room: the so-called patient ribbon, patient companion area, open bathroom, caregiver workstation and caregiver hub. The room incorporates multiple versatile and modular elements, such as the patient ribbon, which collects many of the disparate elements commonly found in healthcare environments into a single, streamlined, patient-centred piece of infrastructure that extends from headwall to footwall. It provides easy access to electrical, technological and gas supply components as well as the patient media centre, which helps facilitate collaboration between caregivers, patients and visitors. It also provides connectivity to entertainment, information and hospital services.

1   The bed and the patient are the centre of attention.

2–3   Changing lighting scenarios

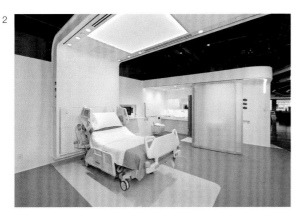

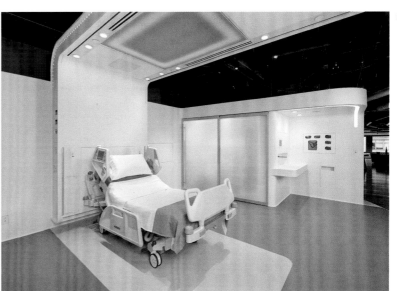

2

3

4 A floor-level shower with coloured glass doors

5 Washbasin with touch-free tap fitting

6 The washbasin is a one-piece moulding made of a mineral-based plastic composite.

7 Technical ports and a digital workstation

8 Integral striplamp

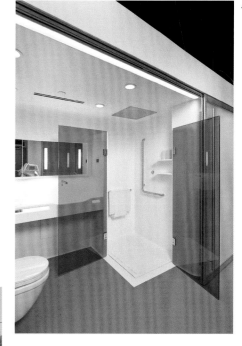

4

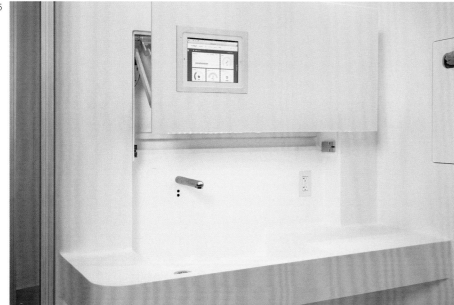

5

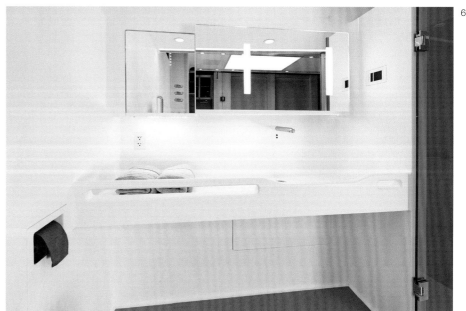

6

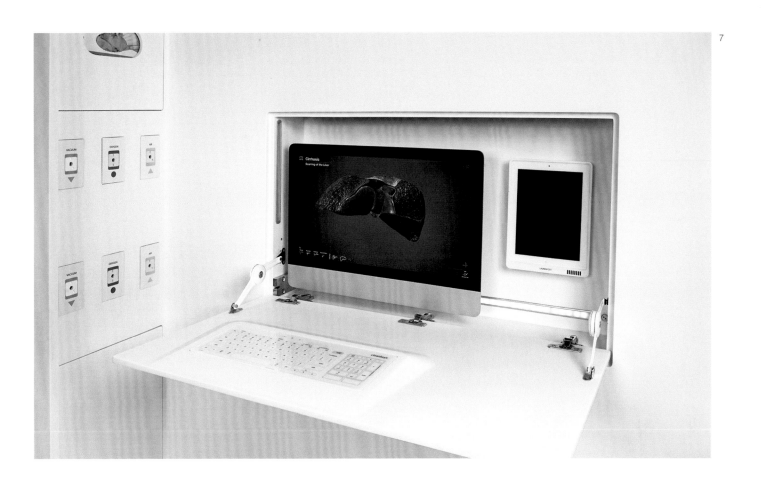

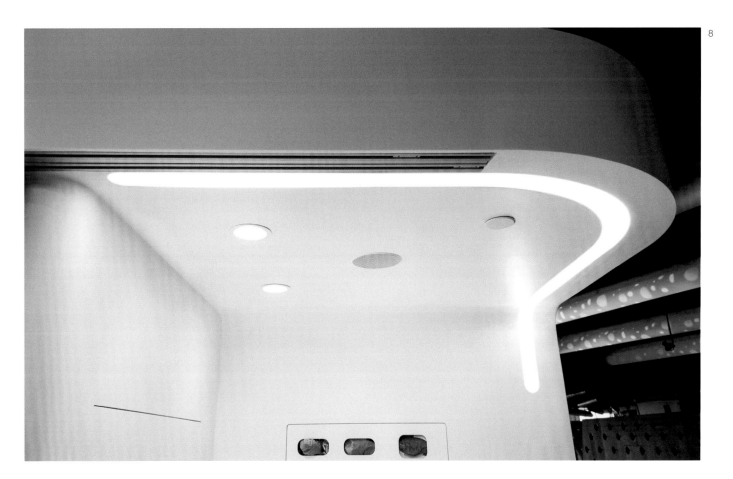

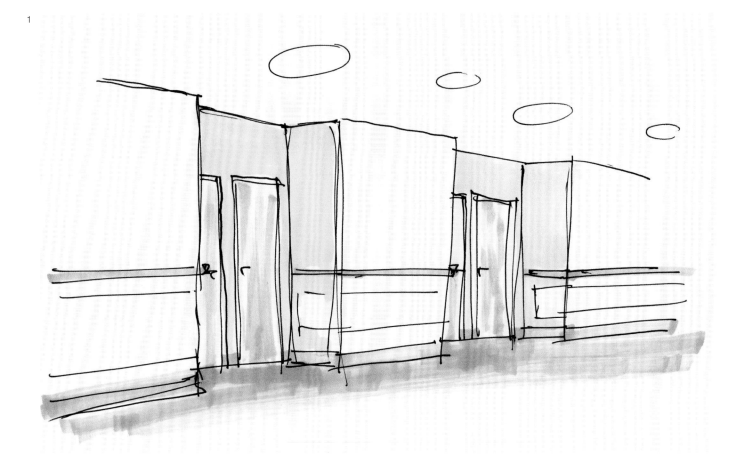

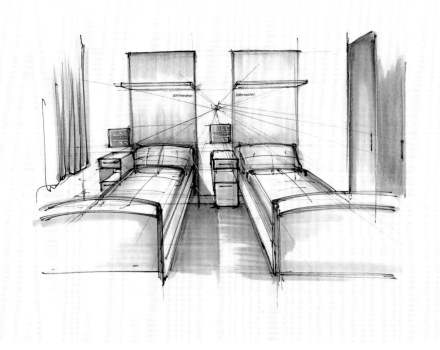

Workflow: planning, interfaces and methods

1   Sketch of a colour
    concept for door niches

2   Sketch of a two-bed
    arrangement

What determines the design of a patient room? A key determinant is the need for a hospital to operate with maximum efficiency – not just in standard day-to-day operations but also in emergency situations. In the planning of new hospitals, simulation tools are therefore used to optimise the paths that staff take, as staff costs are, in most of the world, the single greatest cost factor in hospital operations. The cost-efficient technical organisation of hospitals and hospital rooms is therefore of paramount importance.

Hospital interiors – especially in new hospital buildings – are typically designed by the responsible architecture office together with interior architects (a protected profession in Germany) or interior designers. Alternatively, the design of the hospital

interiors may be commissioned as a separate planning task undertaken by a suitably qualified interior architecture office.

The modernisation or refurbishment of specific hospital interiors, such as individual wards, patient rooms, nursing stations, corridors or lounges is often motivated by a need to keep up with and compete with other healthcare providers. To attract privately-insured patients, hospitals also provide contemporary, modern patient rooms with a hotel-like atmosphere that can be billed as a supplementary service.

In the case of the redesign of existing hospital interiors, the services of an architect may not be required at all. In such cases, a specialist interior architecture

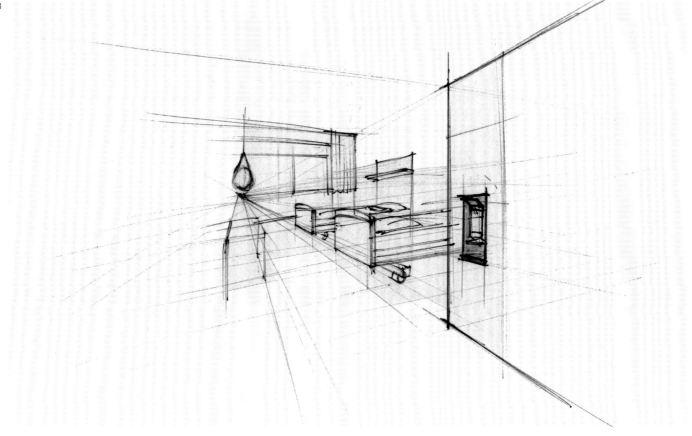

3 Quick perspective sketch of a two-bed arrangement

4 Floor plan of bed wards. a|sh architekten, Siloah-Oststadt-Heide-haus Clinic, Hanover, Germany

5 Luxurious room for psychosomatic patients in a private clinic. 100% interior Sylvia Leydecker, Limes Schlossklinik, Teschow, Germany

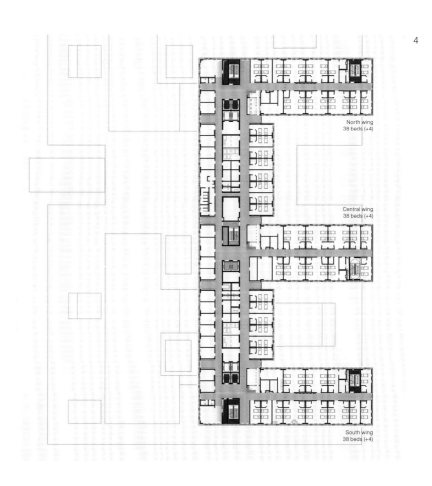

4

North wing
38 beds (+4)

Central wing
38 beds (+4)

South wing
38 beds (+4)

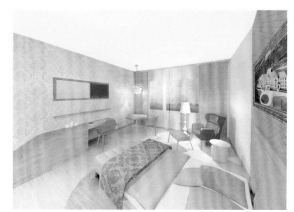

office may work together in a team with the hospital's own in-house technicians or building department.

Working within existing built structures always involves a degree of compromise and adaptation. An interior architect may be tasked with converting multi-bed rooms into two-bed or single-bed rooms, or vice versa, or with removing joint washing facilities in favour of individual bathrooms. A ward may need to be extended or alternatively may just require a cosmetic "make-over". In some cases, interior architects may only be commissioned to design loose furnishings and artworks (DIN 276 cost group 600), to specify furniture or devise a colour and material concept for room surfaces. Similarly, a hospital may decide to upgrade only a few individual rooms in a ward as an interim solution prior to the building of a new wing of premium patient rooms, whereupon the rooms will be returned to a simpler standard.

The interface between architecture and interior architecture

From a business perspective, hospitals will want to achieve the best possible prospect of economic success with the least possible risk. To this end, they put together a team of relevant professionals; interior architects therefore commonly work together with architects and other experts and specialist planners in a team.

There is no set point at which an interior architecture office joins a project. One reason may be that interior architects are only commissioned once the client has learnt the value of their input, and in turn the value of good interior architecture, which can happen at different times in the building process.

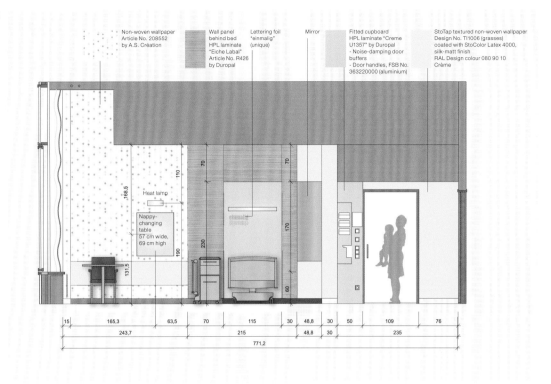

Non-woven wallpaper
Article No. 208552
by A.S. Création

Wall panel
behind bed
HPL laminate
"Eiche Labal"
Article No. R426
by Duropal

Lettering foil
"einmalig"
(unique)

Mirror

Fitted cupboard
HPL laminate "Creme
U1357" by Duropal
- Noise-damping door
buffers
- Door handles, FSB No.
363220000 (aluminium)

StoTap textured non-woven wallpaper
Design No. TI1006 (grasses)
coated with StoColor Latex 4000,
silk-matt finish
RAL Design colour 080 90 10
Crème

Heat lamp

Nappy-
changing
table
57 cm wide,
69 cm high

Interior architects can be involved at a very early stage in a project as part of a feasibility study to determine how realistic a project is and how feasible it is financially. Similarly, interior architects may also be brought in before a project starts to help communicate and visualise the idea with a view to convincing decision makers, for example politicians, to go ahead with the project. The involvement of an interior architecture office at this point is therefore primarily strategic.

Interior architecture can also be considered prior to building works commencing. In such cases, details of surface materials and fittings, such as patient room cupboards, may already be defined long before the rooms are fitted out. The advantage here is that the design of the interiors and the overall architecture can go hand in hand, allowing interior architects to contribute to decisions such as the placement of bathrooms for natural illumination, the design of wayfinding elements or the position and size of windows.

At the latest, the interior design of hospitals should begin when the building plans and/or building shell starts to take form. After a period of

initial preliminary investigations to determine planning parameters, the interior design should proceed swiftly to allow sufficient time for tendering, evaluating and adjusting bids so that the relevant construction trades can begin as soon as building progress allows.

Teamwork, decision-making and collaboration with other experts

Compared with the design of other interiors, for example offices, designing hospital interiors involves numerous participants with different standpoints and priorities, for example the hospital management, medical director, care management, hygiene experts, technical services, the in-house building department, medical and care staff, the facility management office, external consultants brought in to optimise revenues, and so on. While this is enriching, it also complicates processes and makes progress slower. In the frequently highly

7

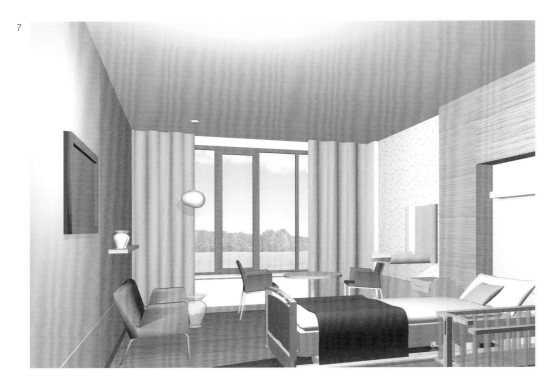

6   Interior wall elevation of a
    premium maternity room.
    100% interior Sylvia Leydecker,
    Rems-Murr Hospital,
    Winnenden, Germany

7   3D visualisation showing the
    interior of a premium maternity
    room. Rems-Murr Hospital

hierarchical organisational structure of hospitals, decision-making is rarely democratic, and ensuring that different standpoints, for example that of staff, are also heard can at times be difficult.

It is invariably necessary to acquaint oneself with the specific structure and dynamics of the group of participants in order to learn which approaches are most effective. A strategic approach coupled with tact and diplomacy and an awareness of personal sensibilities and potential points of resistance go a long way towards reaching one's goals. The respective sensibilities of head doctors and boards of directors need to be taken into account as well as the wishes of staff, input from technical planners, hygiene recommendations or even the involvement of the friends' society. Personal preferences expressed by individual team members are not always so straightforward to incorporate and can complicate reaching a decision. The quality of the interior design concept is therefore just one part of the process; the clever, diplomatic consideration of the different interests of the various participants and stakeholders can be equally vital to achieving a successful result.

The need to reconcile these different interests can at times be a difficult balancing act requiring compromises that individual participants may find unsatisfactory. In addition to professional knowledge and experience, designers therefore also need social competencies, psychological sensitivity as well as diplomatic skills to strategically reach their aims.

Innovative tools such as Computer-Aided Facility Management Systems (CAFM: a computer-aided information system for the strategic and operative coordination of all building management services) are often not available to provide a planning basis. Likewise, reliable information is not always available when designing within existing buildings. In practice, the interior design is therefore often undertaken in conjunction with an architect, or else together with the hospital's in-house technical department.

It can be a difficult and laborious process for all involved. Architects and interior architects are well-advised to work together as sparring partners and team players to jointly champion good design where technocratic and economic concerns otherwise prevail.

Design

The design process is defined by the boundary conditions and key parameters, among them the overall architectural concept, the urban and natural surroundings as well as the current status quo of the respective spaces. Fire safety requirements must be fulfilled and work patterns optimised to maximise process efficiency. At the same time, the design presents an opportunity to re-examine how the hospital sees itself, its image, clinical focus and key patient target groups with a view to clarifying hospital marketing and incorporating facility management.

Aside from practical and functional concerns, the design must align with the scale of services that a hospital bills to the patient or the patient's health insurance. Without this, a redesign is merely a costly exercise for a hospital. It is vitally important to identify the corresponding criteria early in the design process. Better comfort and aesthetic qualities are billable as supplementary services (i.e. not in regular patient rooms), which is why they are of interest to the client.

BIM, fee-paying scales, for example the German HOAI for architectural and engineering services, regulations and standards, such as the DIN norms, as well as planning processes are constantly changing. As hospitals become more international, so too does hospital planning. Innovative planning tools such as BIM improve international collaboration in the design and planning of large-scale projects by providing a central data platform for the exchange of planning information. Organised around the floor plans and room heights, it can store all data necessary for the interior design. A good design results in a well-rounded overall design concept. Aside from the specific design skills, interior architects must have relevant experience in the field of healthcare planning, for example with regard to hygiene requirements and work processes. Starting from a design sketch or working model, the designer develops all aspects of the design for presentation to the client in the form of plans, elevations, sketches, 3D visualisations or even short films that communicate a vision of the resulting interiors. Moodboards can also be used to communicate an intended atmosphere, along with material collages to give a haptic sense of the room and its fittings. A factual written description of the design along with a more marketing-oriented text help communicate the idea to other decision makers.

As the project progresses, a sample room can be particularly effective for evaluating furnishings, for example tables and chairs, or tap fittings, surface qualities and textiles. A full-scale mock-up can be built or an actual room converted as a prototype for evaluation by the team members, making it possible to test the ease of cleaning or resistance of materials to detergents. While a design should reflect as many different perspectives as possible, in practice it is frequently necessary to prioritise certain aspects to arrive at an adequate result. Ideally, the design has reached an advanced stage before a real or mock-up prototype is built, so that all that remains are optimisations and fine-tuning.

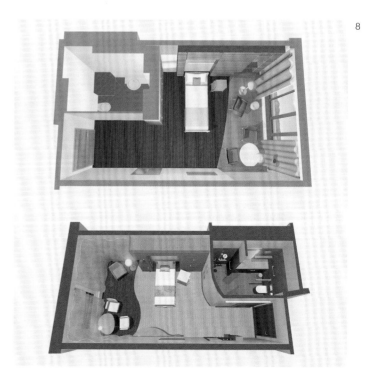

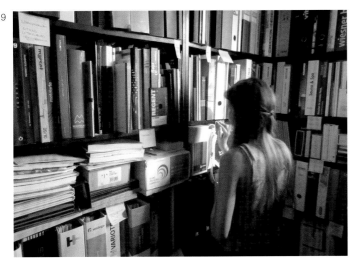

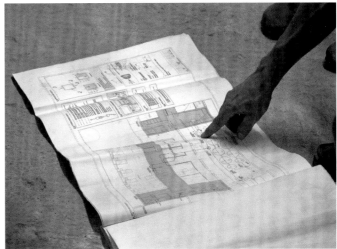

8 Bird's eye view of a premium single
room with bathroom. 100% interior
Sylvia Leydecker, Rems-Murr
Hospital, Winnenden, Germany

9 Researching in the material library of an
interior design office

10 Consulting plans on the construction
site. TAMassociati, Paediatric Centre,
Port Sudan, Sudan

11 Material collage showing the subtle
colour palette in the premium rooms for
psychosomatic patients

12 Model of the patient room of the future

13 Material samples on a conference table

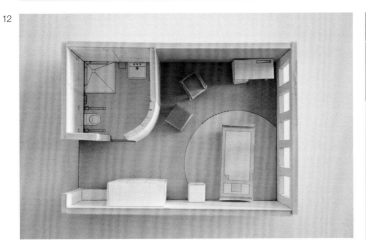

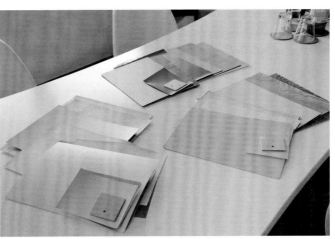

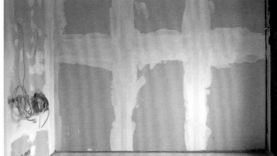

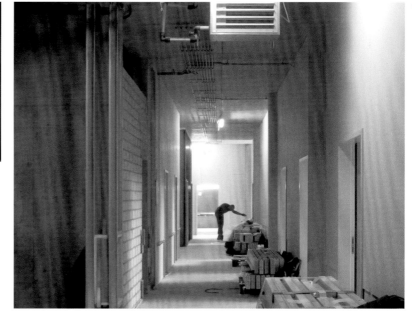

14 Gypsum plasterboard
wall prior to cladding

15 Hospital corridor in
mid-construction

Tendering, bids
and contract awarding

A detailed specification is drawn up based on the design and is then put out to tender. The resulting bids need to be evaluated and bidder interviews conducted before contracts are awarded for construction works. Drawing up specifications can be complex and in the case of large contracts must adhere to statutory tendering procedures. Considerable time and attention is required to comprehensively and precisely specify building works, especially when a particular product, model or product range is envisaged. Manufacturers often supply relevant specification texts to ease this process. Some trades may be awarded individually, others, such as wall and floor coverings, in combination, or all together from a single contractor. The different bids are compared with one another to determine the most economical bid – though this is not necessarily the cheapest. Relevant candidates are then recommended to the client, who will generally conduct one or more rounds of discussions with bidders before awarding the final contract.

In terms of economics, the interior design concept should strive to achieve maximum effect with a minimum input of resources, especially with respect to time and costs. The danger here is that aesthetic concerns may be sidelined in the long and slow process from design to completion, falling victim to hard facts such as time and cost constraints. A successful interior design concept should therefore always pay heed to economic concerns. It is not unusual for further design cuts to be made during the tendering and contract awarding phase, or for cheaper alternatives to be sought. Interior architects should take care to ensure the quality of the room design is upheld.

Even before building works begin, there is always a danger that progress may be delayed for political, financial or technical reasons. Building works must be supervised to ensure that what is built corresponds to the design plans. Refurbishments within an existing building usually make it necessary to conduct works while the hospital is in operation. This is a sensitive area that needs careful planning, particularly with regard to the timing of building works. One should clarify in advance whether it is better to schedule building works vertically or horizontally (for example floor by floor). In either case, all especially noisy construction work, such as the demolition of dividing walls or chiselling off floor tiles should be scheduled to coincide with low occupancy periods in the hospital, such as over public holidays. It may even be advisable to seek an alternative solution, such as the direct application of a filler and a new floor covering.

The building process begins with the bathrooms and installation of services, then the treatment of bounding surfaces such as the floors and walls, including any embedded or recessed lighting, followed by interior fittings such as cupboards, and finally furniture and furnishings. All this needs to be supervised during construction and assessed on completion, remedying any remaining problems as necessary. Only then are the rooms handed over to the users and patients, with the design hopefully contributing to a constant bed occupancy rate.

Cost and time constraints are often prioritised over aesthetic concerns. The supervising interior architect should therefore be watchful to ensure corners are not cut. Costs are monitored with every step of the building process, from the initial estimate to the cost calculations and final cost statement. However, some building projects separate design and project management into two separate tasks from the outset, with the latter often undertaken by the hospital's technical department.

If, as building works near completion, financial resources start to run short, cost savings may be implemented that can impact on the interior design as one of the final stages of the building construction. This is, however, often short-sighted as it affects an area that patients experience most directly, along with meals, and on which they base their assessment of the quality of a hospital, and by implication of its medical services.

On completion of building works, the facility is handed over to the client who will invariably conduct an assessment of the work executed prior to use. Any functional or aesthetic defects should ideally be remedied before patient rooms and associated areas are occupied by the first patients. Differences of opinion at this late stage, especially concerning the remedying of defects, can cause major inconvenience and may even lead to legal proceedings. Liability aspects may mean that rooms cannot be used, and a protracted stand-off can cause contractors to become insolvent. It is therefore advisable to anticipate potential problems in advance to find a timely resolution. In most cases, however, patient rooms will be declared fit for use, and can be put into service. A good design is usually reflected by a consistently high bed occupancy rate.

BIM

In future planning processes, BIM looks set to become a suitable tool for international cooperation as it allows all members of the design team to work simultaneously on a project by referencing data stored in the cloud. Instead of drawing in 2D, models are constructed in 3D. BIM models also store additional information about the construction, such as time schedules and costs, ensuring ongoing project transparency and making it possible to monitor and control the progress of the project across all phases of the building process. Aside from the initial cost of investment, data interface problems and data security are two critical areas for which solutions are needed.

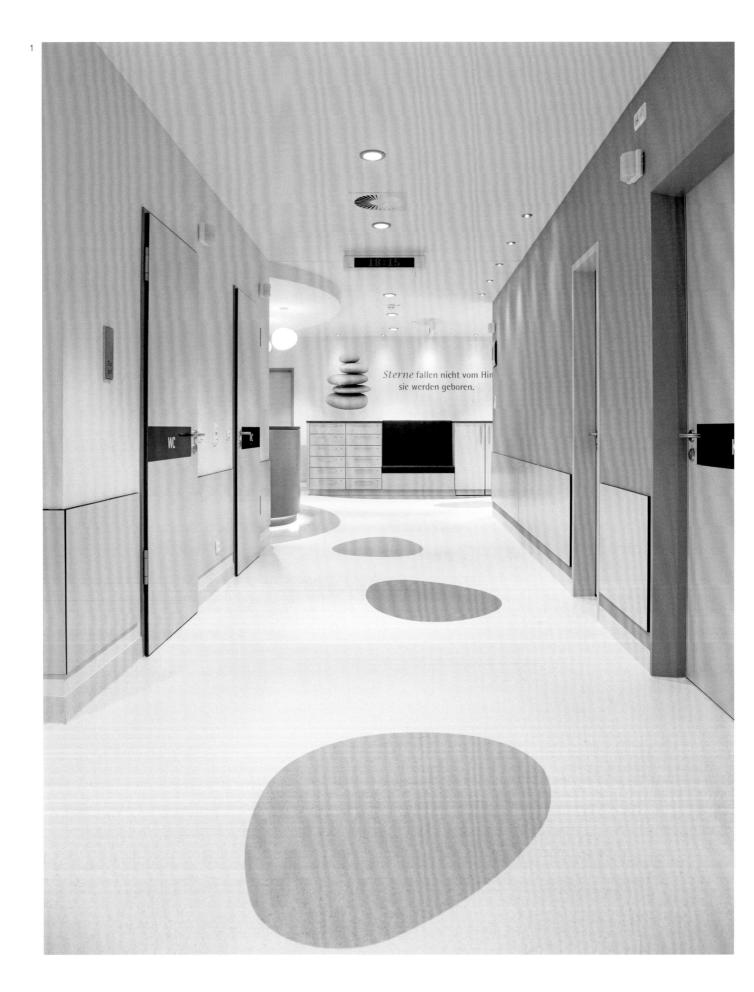

Business economics, marketing and operations

1   A high-quality medical facility
    with wellness character reduces
    stress for patients and staff alike.
    100% interior Sylvia Leydecker,
    St. Elisabeth Hospital, Essen,
    Germany

Aside from creating a more patient-centred environment, every investment in interior design must ultimately also deliver a return on investment, and offer something of additional value.

In Germany, medical and healthcare services are billed on a per-case basis according to so-called Diagnosis Related Groups (DRGs). Since their introduction, the time patients spend in hospital has decreased, as has the number of beds, while the number of cases has increased. Well-designed interiors that promote patient well-being improve the speed of recovery and decrease the time spent in hospital, improving patient turnaround, which is good for revenue. In practice, however, the benefit is minimal as patients are discharged early anyway. In the USA, the Patient Protection and Affordable Care Act (PPACA, introduced by Barack Obama in 2010 and known popularly as "Obamacare", which provides access to healthcare for social groups without private health insurance) has led to a significant rise in the number of outpatient facilities, effecting a shift from inpatient to outpatient care, and with it a greater focus on prevention.

The pressure to save costs in the healthcare sector means that budgets are frequently constrained. Cost-effective planning in the context of architecture is therefore about achieving a good balance between costs and revenue by optimising processes, incorporating hygiene requirements and using affordable means for modularity and flexibility. In hospital planning, technocratic thinking, organisational concerns and cost-efficiency remain the primary dictates. Indeed, public health legislation requires that hospitals operate efficiently (in Germany stipulated in §12 SGB 5 – Volume 5 of the German Social Code), and that chosen measures be sufficient and appropriate and not beyond what is necessary. The key question here is what is sufficient to keep up with other competitors and to remain competitive in the future.

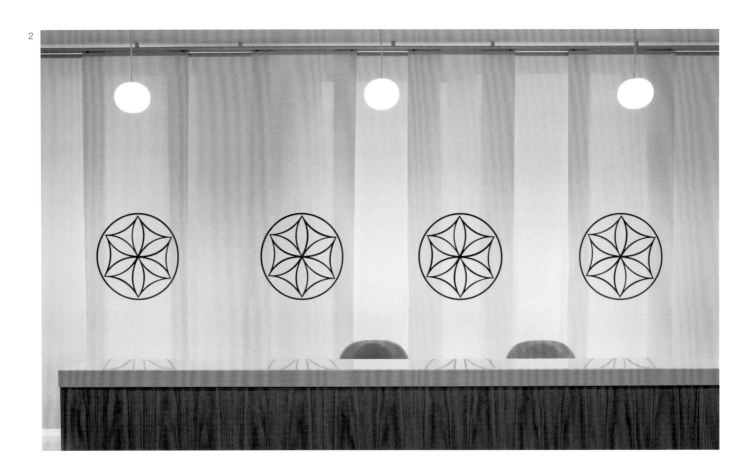

If interior design is understood as a strategic means of successfully establishing a position in the healthcare market, its contribution to the creation of value becomes immediately apparent. Part of this strategy is that the quality of hospital stays matches the target group and overall vision.

Quality and cost-effectiveness are not mutually exclusive. On the contrary, they condition one another. Better occupancy rates, i.e. an increase in case numbers, can be achieved through better-quality interior design. Interior architecture brings economic benefits when a better standard of design actually improves the quality of hospital stays.

Widespread economisation in the healthcare sector focusses attention on the ratio between costs and revenue. Typically, revenue optimisation is achieved on the one hand by minimising costs and on the other by increasing efficiency. More efficient

services result in greater throughput and greater revenue. In some cases, however, this has resulted in an economically-motivated over-provision of services, for example inpatient treatment where outpatient care may suffice, or even medical procedures that are not strictly necessary. In the USA, the Choosing Wisely initiative (www.choosingwisely.org) founded by the National Physicians Alliance has been monitoring and campaigning against this problem in the healthcare sector for years.

Staff

Personnel costs are the single greatest cost factor in hospital operations, and the hospital design and architecture should help ensure that staff resources are used as effectively as possible. In addition, shortages of skilled staff among both

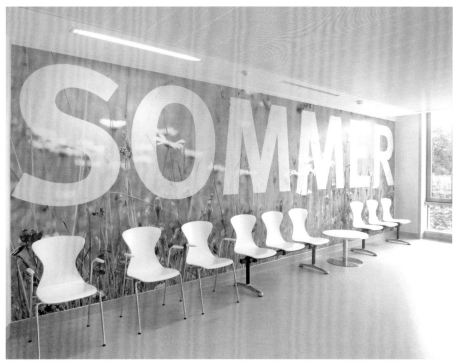

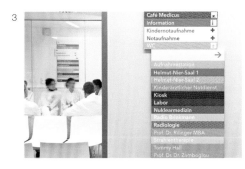

medical personnel and carers mean that there is increasing competition to attract staff. Nursing staff and carers are also poorly paid and subject to high stress levels resulting from the heavy workload and pressure to work efficiently, which contributes to the profession's overall negative image. To retain staff, hospitals need to provide working environments that contribute to a better work-life balance: rest rooms that allow staff to properly relax, take a break and gain new strength and energy; pleasant hospital environments that help rather than hinder work processes, that communicate a sense of value in their work and make their work tolerable and worthwhile. The interior architecture can therefore be a tangible factor in the competition for qualified staff. An attractive and functional workplace that is well-designed and pleasant to be in, and reflects the value of the work undertaken, can be a decisive aspect in the choice of employer. Such workplaces should enable work to proceed smoothly through a sensible arrangement of paths and spaces, and minimise noise levels through suitable acoustic design to decrease environment-induced stress. Similarly, measures that improve the ergonomics of the workplace, such as sufficiently wide openings, adequate space to move around, sensible equipment heights and so on, as well as haptic and visual cues can also help to significantly reduce stress levels at work. Finally, interiors should communicate a sense of identity that can serve as a psychological anchor, helping staff to value their specific workplace and acquire a sense of belonging. This is especially important in large, sprawling hospital complexes.

Good healthcare interiors contribute to the process of healing and recovery and to the effective operation of a ward, reducing the incidence of costly staff absences due to physical or psychological illness.

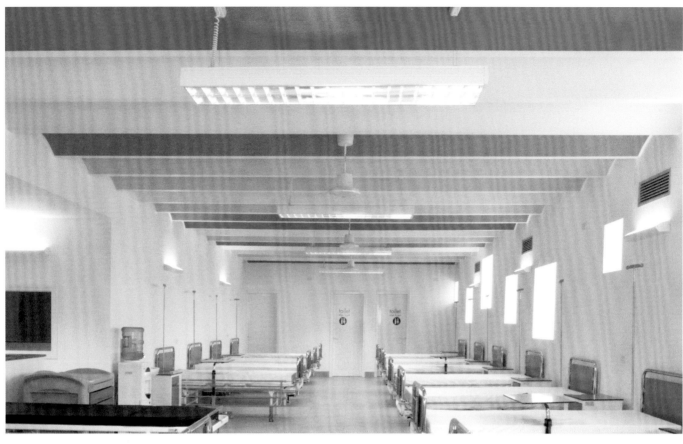

Corporate interiors

The elaboration of a corporate identity (CI) that
reflects the soul and values of a hospital and its
specific approach is the basis for finding an overall
formal design language. It is commonly expressed
in the corporate design of the hospital's marketing
collateral such as the logo, website and brochure.
This two-dimensional principle is sometimes carried
over in a half-hearted manner to the hospital interiors through the application of logos on textiles or
door mats, or posters in hospital corridors. A more
effective approach to corporate interiors, on the
other hand, is three-dimensional and reflects the
brand values and character of the hospital as manifested in the choice of materials, colours and forms.

A coherent CI therefore serves as the basis for
the design of corporate interiors. Wayfinding
systems and signage can potentially play a key

role in defining the character of interiors; however, all too often, they do not relate to the actual
architecture of the interiors, and fail to contribute
to its atmosphere.

Corporate interiors are part of a strategic marketing tool that should be applied consistently across
all media. Based on an analysis of the existing
situation and a vision for the future, the marketing
concept should therefore also encompass the spatial characteristics of the hospital. This is typically
experienced at two levels: the patient's experience
of the corporate interiors and the overall corporate
architecture of the hospital.

A coherent and convincing corporate design concept operates at all levels, as per the principle that
"you cannot not communicate". Ideally, as patients
and users experience the hospital, the corporate
design reinforces the institution's unique charac-

6

5   A multi-bed room, if comfort-
    able, can also meet patient
    expectations in some contexts.
    TAMassociati, Paediatric Centre,
    Port Sudan, Sudan

6   In this luxury hospital in a castle,
    the reception for privately-health-
    insured patients is a mixture of
    Baroque and carefully selected
    contemporary designer-kitsch.
    100% interior Sylvia Leydecker,
    Limes Schlossklinik, Teschow,
    Germany

ter and approach. A good interior design has the fantastic potential to make the experience of being in hospital a memorable and positive experience. It strengthens the positive public perception of the hospital and by implication also of its services.

Marketing for specific target groups

A successful corporate interior strengthens the hospital brand both outwardly and inwardly, reinforcing faith in the medical competency of its staff and creating a sense of personal identification for the patient as well as for the employee. From a patient's perspective, the profile of a hospital reflects on the quality of its medical care. Well-designed interiors that communicate a sense of security and a feeling of being looked after help to reduce anxiety and

reinforce trust. The image that patients and visitors associate with the quality of the interior is in turn applied to the quality of medical care.

For staff, a good corporate interior strengthens their sense of identity and belonging, in turn motivating them to act accordingly. Positive public opinion can likewise lend weight to the position of politics, which is continually being questioned from all sides. It also has an effect on referring doctors and health insurance providers. The interior architecture as an indicator of quality therefore helps hospitals acquire a market advantage and improve profitability. And this is what a hospital ultimately needs to achieve to continue successfully treating and healing people.

Building a successful hospital brand takes time and money. It must be elaborated continually and coherently to establish sufficient brand visibility.

From then on, the process of forming, adjusting and promoting the brand is an ongoing process. Constant brand revisions that lack a clear strategy or direction make little sense both in material terms and economically. A strong, vibrant brand, on the other hand, reflects the agility of a hospital and its ability to position itself and remain independent as circumstances change. Rooms aimed at specific target groups are no exception to this rule.

Billing services

The economic viability of a hospital depends on providing defined billable services. Some health insurers remunerate on a performance basis (pay for performance, P4P) whereby payment is made for meeting defined performance measures. However this also means that no money is paid if performance measures are not met. A needs-based financing method is therefore essential.

The design of premium patient rooms for patients with private health insurance must fulfil certain criteria. A comfortable, well-designed patient room is a supplementary bookable option that, along with other comfort options such as special culinary provisions, incurs an extra charge. For German private health insurers, a hospital's premium rooms must differ sufficiently from the regular patient rooms to qualify as a supplementary option. Hospitals that improve their regular patient rooms may therefore be at a disadvantage as they are not able to bill for as many supplementary services. Relevant criteria include whether the patient room is a single-bed or a two-bed room, the size of the bathroom, the position and view from the room, and so on. Privately-insured patients expect a more hotel-like atmosphere as manifested in the appearance of the materials and a better level of comfort, for example through lighting options or comfortable furnishings. A tasteful, high-quality hotel atmosphere optimised to meet private health insurance criteria therefore pays off.

Ideally, everyone should be able to benefit from good patient room design. At present, however, this is restricted to patients with private health insurance, as it is not a billable aspect of regular healthcare services.

Durability and hospital operations

In the case of both new buildings and existing building conversions, of primary concern is the cost of investment. However, lifecycle costs are also equally relevant, not least because cumulative hospital running costs, on average, exceed the initial investment costs after seven years. The maintenance costs of materials, constructions and products, along with operating costs such as electricity, water, cleaning and repairs, must therefore also be considered during the initial design process.

Once the rooms are completed, focus shifts to the functional durability of the products and materials used. The need to repair or replace items or equipment not only costs money but can also result in service outages that can likewise be costly and should be considered in advance during the planning process.

Damaged chairs, sofas or benches create a negative impression, and worn or torn upholstery additionally represents a hygiene risk. If not remedied, the situation will persist with potentially grave consequences. A resulting loss of patient trust is damaging to business and, as such, there is no good economic reason for not effecting repairs. Outmoded hospital interiors are usually, therefore, the product of an ongoing lack of investment. Occasionally, financing problems during the planning process, which can have all manner of causes, may cause projects to stall, sometimes even delaying completion for several years.

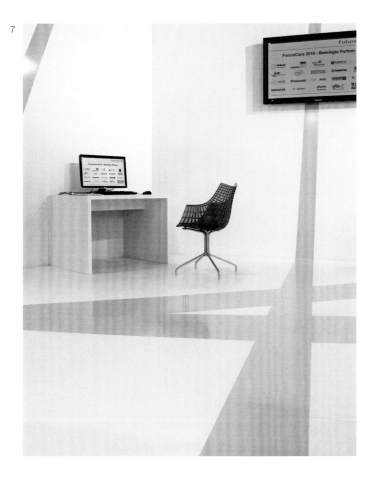

7 Advances in digitisation will make rooms smarter, interactive and networked with the help of IT and sensor technology. 100% interior Sylvia Leydecker, FutureCare 2010, CeBIT, Hanover, Germany

Hospital 4.0 and upholding the human perspective

Digitised patient rooms and smart hospitals are just around the corner. The "green hospital", which, in addition to being smart, aims to be sustainable and environmentally-friendly, is likewise the subject of intensive research and development. As energy costs rise and eclipse material costs, ecological principles gain increasing relevance. Personnel costs, too, remain a significant economic factor; in addition, staff are burdened with ever-increasing tasks of documentation, a tendency that encroaches on the quality of service. IT costs also rise exponentially each year, and hospitals now lag significantly behind other industries. The implementation costs and effort required to switch and update systems is such that health providers apply these across several hospitals at once to maximise synergy effects and economies of scale.

Digital systems can notify when maintenance is necessary and show the location of equipment for better and more effective facility management, thereby reducing maintenance costs. Smart energy concepts can help reduce energy consumption. Interior architecture can contribute here by using energy-efficient LEDs or OLEDs, or smart materials such as latent heat accumulators (PCMs), which also help to reduce day-to-day energy consumption. Similarly, the use of innovative materials such as anti-bacterial or anti-soiling coatings and easy-to-clean or self-cleaning photocatalytic surfaces can reduce cleaning costs.

In future, the design of patient rooms will incorporate sensors and controller technology, for example in lighting or tap fittings. Optimisations in interfaces between different systems such as lighting or media technology, or the intelligent networking of different hospital functions using polymer optical fibres (POF) will improve functionality and make equipment simpler to use. Robots are already used to transport containers around hospitals, and new robots are being tested for use in wards to automate routine tasks and reduce staff workload. In future, they may also represent an economical alternative to resolving staff shortages.

Hospital 4.0 will generate increasing quantities of data including data on patients, which health insurance providers, among others, will want to access for a widening array of purposes – much like their counterparts in the online world, who already monitor our consumer preferences. Data protection regulations currently restrict this, although some argue that this is holding back progress and advances in technology. As with any new technology, however, the benefits and risks need to be weighed up against each other. For many it would seem that comfort, convenience and the economic benefits outweigh the need for data protection.

In 2018, a new EU Data Protection Directive will come into force to help protect and regulate access to sensitive data and will likely have implications for the linking of intelligent systems in hospital interiors. Today, data protection concerns can already be addressed in the design of hospital interiors through the arrangement of the reception, patient admission area and nursing stations. All these areas must observe patient privacy concerns, for example by ensuring that sensitive consultations take place in acoustically separated areas. In a hospital, the level of personal privacy is inherently compromised, and here too interior architecture can contribute by improving the degree of private sphere for patients and providing spaces for staff when not on duty.

Sustainability

In contrast to popular opinion, sustainability is not solely about energy efficiency. While the concept of the "green hospital" gained popularity several years ago, it remains largely a contradiction in terms because hospitals necessarily consume vast quantities of energy and medication residues pollute the environment. Nevertheless, environmental certification labels such as LEED, BREEAM and the German DGNB label remain popular among investors, even though some hospitals find the certification procedure too expensive, despite costing a fraction of the overall building costs. For the design of environmentally-friendly hospital interiors, common criteria include the use of environmentally-safe and non-toxic products and materials along with sufficient natural illumination and social facilities such as rest rooms. Products that are environmentally-friendly, for example in their production, are increasingly being specified and also represent a marketing factor. This will require flexible structures, and the ability to develop and adapt to meet new developments in the future.

To summarise, designing for staff and patients always entails finding a balance between numbers, functions and emotions. Personal care and attention and efficiency-enhancing technologies are just as sustainable as the use of environmentally-friendly and recyclable materials made with minimal resources. Ecology and economics can go hand in hand.

A carefully conceived, forward-looking interior design concept that unites general know-how and expertise in the healthcare sector will need to identify which aspects are most important to implement and which are perhaps not as essential as initially thought, also in terms of cost-effectiveness. Interior design concepts that carefully consider the qualities of a space and that are also time- and cost-efficient in their approach have the potential to simultaneously address the aims of optimising revenue, protecting the environment, promoting modern medicine and creating a good-quality healing environment, with everything that entails.

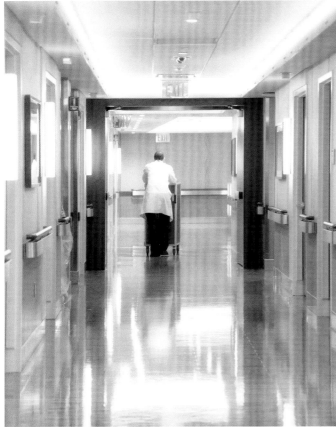

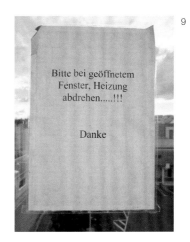

8 People move around in the highly technological medicinal environments of modern hospitals. e4h architecture, Lenox Hill Hospital, New York, USA

9 "Turn down the heating when you open the window" – Energy efficiency in 2016. In future, smart controls will take care of this.

10 The patient between technology and nature. HPP Architekten, Olgahospital and Gynaecological Clinic, Stuttgart, Germany

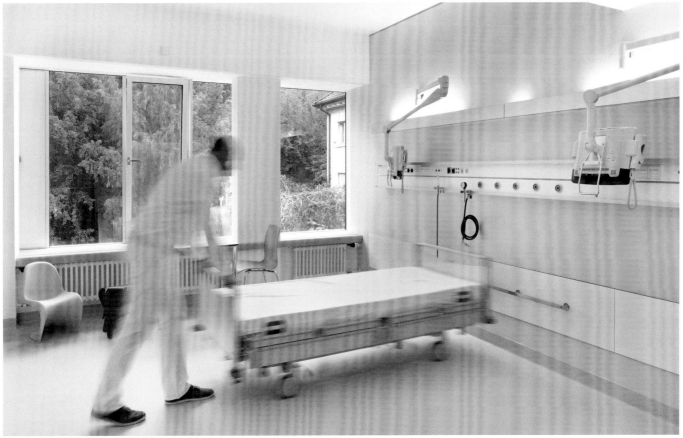

10

Acknowledgements

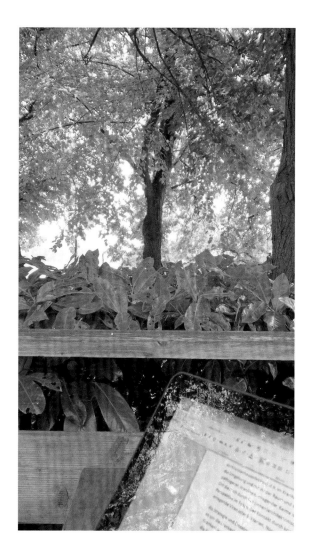

The "making of" this book is the work of a team of committed people, all of whom have contributed their part. In my work as an author, as well as in my chosen profession, that of an interior architect, I spend most of my time "on the front line". Without my "crew" to back me up, this book would not have existed, or at least not in this quality.

I would like to thank all those who played a part in its fruition:

My colleagues in the profession who supported the idea I floated at a congress on the topic, and my publisher, Birkhäuser Verlag, for responding so positively to my book proposal.

I would like to thank the many offices around the world who supplied me with information on their projects along with images, a selection of which can be seen in the book. Some of them I knew already, and some I have grown to know and cherish over the course of researching for this book. The research proved to be both stimulating and challenging as, in many cases, the patient room was only rarely the focus of the respective projects.

I had excellent support from the publisher's team through all phases of the book, from the editing and translation to layout and production to distribution and marketing. In particular, I would like to thank my long-standing editor at Birkhäuser Verlag, Andreas Müller, with whom I started the project, and his colleague Henriette Mueller-Stahl in Berlin for her support and collaboration in completing the project. I would also like to thank Julia Ess for her invaluable support, and Katja Jaeger for her work on the book production. Special thanks also go to Rein Steger, our graphic designer in Barcelona, for the magnificent collaboration. And finally, I would like to thank my translator, Julian Reisenberger in Weimar, who has once again wonderfully captured my informal writing style in his translation.

In my own office, I also have a helpful crew who keep a keen eye on project progress: Julia Küppers, Theresa Scholl, Britta Schumacher, Benedikt Bachler and my daughter Eileen, who undertook multiple virtual trips around the world to meticulously and competently resolve the logistics of the projects.

Thank you, too, to the member of staff at the venerable "Die Krone" Hotel in the Rheingau for providing me with the perfect place to write the introduction with a view of my beloved River Rhine. My thanks, too, to the sponsors who, through their committed support, have helped make this book possible.

It was a pleasure for me to conceive, write and assemble the contents of this book and, last but not least, to bring it to a point where I can release it into the outside world. My hope now is that it can, in turn, contribute to improving the design of patient rooms and to raise the quality of life so that patients can recover more swiftly, and medical and nursing staff have a better work environment. In short, the book is intended as a source of information and inspiration for architects and interior designers as well as for hospital management, so that they can put this aim into practice.

The work we do – whether in a hospital, in the designing of interiors or the production of a book – is always people-focussed. A whole team of committed people has contributed in no small part to the development of this book to provide you, the reader, with what is hopefully an inspiring result.

As the interior architect Eileen Gray once said, "the future projects light, the past only shadows". The same can be said for patient rooms. You're just like a dream.

Sylvia Leydecker
Cologne, Germany, March 2017

About the authors

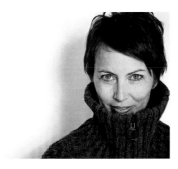

SYLVIA LEYDECKER
Dipl. Ing. Interior Architect BDIA AKG
Sylvia Leydecker is one of Germany's foremost interior architects with specialist expertise in the fields of healthcare, office design, branding and innovative materials. She is director of the studio 100% Interior in Cologne, Germany, specialising in the design of corporate interiors. In the healthcare sector, she works primarily for hospitals and private healthcare facilities, and designed the prototype for a premium patient's room for the Association of Private Health Insurers in Germany (PKV) as well as the FutureCare special exhibition at the CeBit trade fair for the digital association Bitkom.

She studied interior architecture in Wiesbaden, Germany, and at Trisakti University in Jakarta, Indonesia. Before embarking on her creative career, she worked internationally for Deutsche Lufthansa and lived for a while in Manchester, United Kingdom, and Paris, France. She serves in a voluntary capacity as Vice-President of the BDIA Association of German Interior Architects/Designers and was previously a board member of the IFI International Federation of Interior Architects/Designers.

Last but not least, she is the author and editor of several international books on designing interior architecture, corporate interiors and the use of nanomaterials in architecture. Her work as an interior architect and as an author feed into each other, and she takes a conceptual and forward-looking approach to all she does.

PD Dr. med. GEORG DAESCHLEIN
Born in 1959 in Berlin, Germany. Both parents doctors, his father a dermatologist and medical director of Berlin-Neukölln Public Health Department. Georg Daeschlein studied medicine in Berlin and Kiel, Germany, completing his state examination and acquiring his licence to practice medicine in 1985 in Berlin. He is approved as a specialist for laboratory medicine, medical microbiology and infection epidemiology, hygiene and environmental medicine, and dermatology and venereology. In 2011, he completed a post-doctorate in hygiene and environmental medicine. In 2003, he joined the Dermatology Clinic at the University of Greifswald, Germany (Director: Prof. Dr. M. Jünger). Alongside his work at the clinic, he conducts research into preventing the spread of infections and hospital hygiene.

ALAN DILANI
Professor Alan Dilani, Ph.D., is a founder of the International Academy for Design and Health (IADH) and the journal "World Health Design". He holds a Master of Architecture in Environmental Design from the Polytechnic of Turin, Italy, and a Ph.D. in Health Facility Design from the Royal Institute of Technology, Stockholm, Sweden. His multidisciplinary approach to research at the Karolinska Institutet Medical University in Sweden led to a new definition called "Salutogenic Design". He has designed all types of healthcare facilities and has been consulted as an advisor for several ministries of health around the world. He lectures widely and has authored numerous publications. In 2010, Dr Dilani was awarded an AIA Academy of Architecture for Health Award from the American Institute of Architects.

Illustration credits

100% interior Sylvia Leydecker
8, 11 (4, 5), 13 (8), 18, 19 (16, 17), 26 (2), 30, 31 (7, 8),
37 (18), 38 (20, 22), 44, 46 (3), 49 (6), 50 (9), 51 (11),
53 (14), 54 (19), 58 (22), 63, 66 (1), 71 (9, 10), 72/73
(11), 76, 79 (4, 5), 80 (7), 81 (9), 83 (14), 84 (15, 16),
95 (6, 8), 96 (10), 99 (2nd row, 4th ill.), 118 (1, 2),
119 (3, 4, 5), 136 (5, 6), 148 (1, 2), 150 (3), 151, 152,
153, 154, 155 (9, 11, 12, 13), 156 (14, 15), 161 (4),
163, 167 (9), 168

100% interior Sylvia Leydecker; Hessmann, Karin
(photographer)
6, 13 (7, 9, 10), 15 (11), 17, 43, 51 (12), 58 (24), 60,
75, 78 (2, 3), 80 (6), 81 (10), 83 (13), 86, 89 (19, 20),
98, 160, 165

100% interior Sylvia Leydecker; Rosendahl,
Reinhard (photographer)
11 (2), 46 (2), 53 (15), 54 (17), 58 (23), 62 (29),
65, 66 (2, 3), 71 (7, 8), 73 (12), 82 (12), 85, 90 (2),
99 (4th row, 1st ill.), 134, 135 (2, 3), 136 (4),
137 (7, 8, 9, 10), 158, 169

AKAA/Cemal Emden
99 (4th row, 2nd ill.), 138, 139 (2, 3), 140 (5), 141 (7, 8)

© Blunt, Ron (photographer) / www.ronbluntphoto.com
23 (21), 34 (14, 15), 42 (28)

Bonfanti, Marcello © www.marcelbon.com
(photographer)
95 (7)

Borgmann, Roland (photographer)
31 (9)

CallisonRTKL Inc.
12, 20 (19), 99 (1st row, 1st ill.), 100, 101, 102,
103 (4, 5, 6)

Clarke, Peter (photographer)
35 (17), 54 (18)

Cohrssen, Jimmy (photographer)
61 (26, 27)

d2 dintelmann digital (photographer)
20 (18), 39

dwp
24, 62 (28), 92 (4), 99 (3rd row, 2nd ill.), 124, 125,
126 (3, 4), 127 (5, 6, 7, 8, 9)

Friends + Pflaumer Studio GmbH (photographer)
74 (14)

Gollings, John
38 (21)

Grimaldi, Massimo (photographer)
56

Grunert-Held, Ronald (photographer)
68, 69 (5, 6), 74 (13)

© Hamilton Knight, Martine (photographer)
131 (4)

Hein, Tobias, Berlin (photographer)
47

Heinle, Wischer und Partner
107 (5), 105 (2)

HKS, Inc./Blake Marvin
99 (2nd row, 3rd ill.), 114, 115, 116, 117 (4, 5)

Innenarchitektur Thöne
99 (4th row, 3rd ill.), 142 (1, 2), 143 (3, 4)

Karpf, Thorsten (photographer), concept and design:
Bernd Kirchbrücher, raumlinq GmbH
52

Kirchner, Jens (photographer)
35 (16)

Kleiner, Tom (photographer)
28, 32 (10, 11, 12, 13), 82 (11)

Körner, Andreas (photographer)
23 (22, 23), 90 (1), 161 (3)

Landes, Hans Jürgen (photographer)
41 (25, 26)

LUKAS HUNEKE PHOTOGRAPHY (photographer)
26 (3, 4)

Maggie's Centre
129, 130

Malagamba, Duccio
99 (2nd row, 1st ill.), 108, 109

Mariotti, Letizia (photographer)
51 (10), 99 (3rd row, 4th ill.), 132 (1, 2),
133 (3, 4), 167 (8)

Mørk, Adam (photographer)
49 (5, 8)

NBBJ/Airhart, Sean
21, 92 (5)

NBBJ/Dzikowski, Francis/Esto
99 (3rd row, 1st ill.), 120, 121, 122 (3, 4), 123

NBBJ/Griffith, Tim
40, 92 (3)

NXT Health Patient Room 2020 prototype; photo
DuPont™ Corian®, all rights reserved
15 (12), 99 (4th row, 4th ill.), 144, 145 (2, 3),
146 (4, 5, 6), 147 (7, 8)

Pantaleo, Raul (photographer)
162

Reiher, Wolfgang
99 (1st row, 2nd ill.), 104, 105 (3), 106, 107 (6)

Rota, Alesandro (photographer)
11 (3), 96 (9)

sander.hofrichter architekten GmbH Gesellschaft für
Architektur und Generalplanung
112 (4), 113 (9), 150 (4)

sander.hofrichter architekten GmbH Gesellschaft für
Architektur und Generalplanung;
© fotodesign Wolfgang Fallier 99 (2nd row 2nd ill.), 110
(1, 2), 111, 112 (5, 6, 7), 113 (8, 10)

sander.hofrichter architekten GmbH Gesellschaft für
Architektur und Generalplanung; samba-
photography Markus Bachmann (photographer)
81 (8)

© 2016 Stöbe Architekten GmbH & Co. KG;
Martin Schmüdderich, 2012 (photographer)
15 (13)

Spoering, Uwe (photographer)
57

Steinprinz, Sigurd (photographer)
167 (10)

Stüber, Jochen (photographer)
42 (29)

TAF, Gabriella Gustafson & Mattias Ståhlbom;
Åke E:son Lindman (photographer)
37 (19), 41 (27), 49 (7)

TAMassociati
140 (4, 6), 141 (9), 155 (10)

Young, Nigel (photographer)
99 (3rd row, 3rd ill.), 128, 131 (5)

"The greatest enemy of quality is haste."

Henry Ford

DEUTSCHE STEINZEUG AGROB **BUCHTAL**

AGROB BUCHTAL architectural ceramics: symbiosis of functionality and aesthetics

In buildings of the public health service, careful material selection and application are essential for an agreeable ambience supporting the healing process. Wall and floor coverings play a particularly important part there, as they have a significant influence on the functional value and the room atmosphere. According to the relevant studies and findings, forms, surfaces, textures and colours are decisive psychological aspects in this context. As a competent supplier of architectural ceramics, AGROB BUCHTAL offers creative possibilities such as e.g. the modular tile systems ChromaPlural or Emotion for their implementation in practice. They permit the realisation of comprehensive and individual concepts, and that in the long term: even in case of extreme exposure to light and intensive cleaning, there are no gradual or even abrupt changes in colour. Further design options are provided by collections with representative tiles up to the format of 60x120 cm, which convey an impression of sovereign elegance in XXL size.

However, not only the aesthetic but also the functional values are convincing: special non-slip surfaces permit a differentiated slip resistance in the sanitary area of patient rooms and ensure safe walking even when wet. The well-known advantages of ceramic wall and floor coverings are further enhanced by the HT ("Hydrophilic Tile") coating durably baked onto the glaze already in the factory. Following the principle of the photocatalysis, this innovative solution is activated by natural or artificial light and lends ceramic tiles of AGROB BUCHTAL special characteristics: they are extremely easy to clean, have an antibacterial effect without using chemical products and eliminate unwelcome odours as well as air pollutants. All of these advantages come in useful every day and contribute to an improvement of comfort and quality of life.

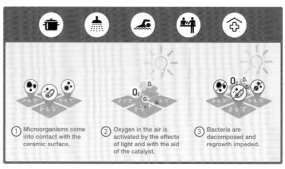

① Microorganisms come into contact with the ceramic surface.
② Oxygen in the air is activated by the effects of light and with the aid of the catalyst.
③ Bacteria are decomposed and regrowth impeded.

HT coating of AGROB BUCHTAL: antibacterial effect without using chemical products

In this sanitary area of a patient room larger tile formats are combined with a filigree ceramic mosaic to discreetly indicate different zones of use and to create a subtle, unobtrusive charm - an intention which is also supported by the colours.

Tiles of AGROB BUCHTAL with HT coating are marked with this logo.

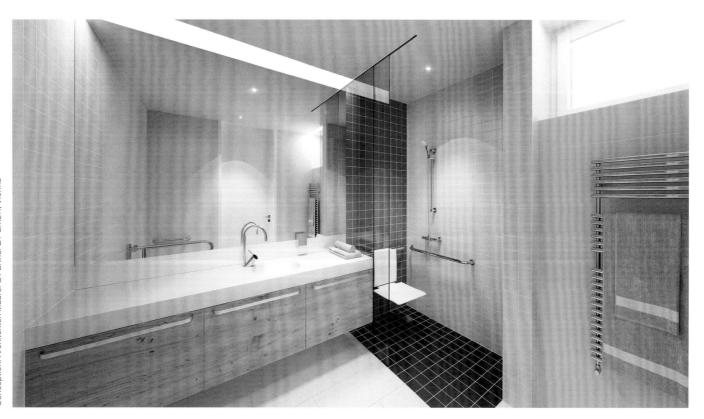

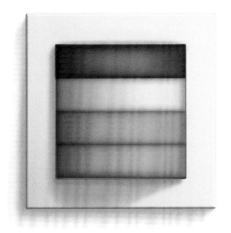
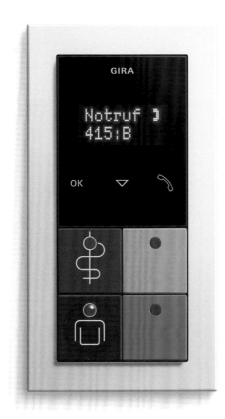
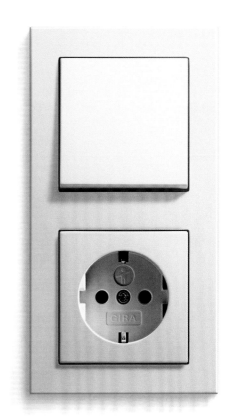
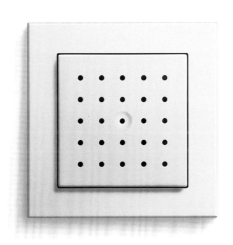

GIRA

Intelligent
Building Technology
since 1905

Gira Giersiepen GmbH & Co. KG (www.gira.com) based in Radevormwald is one of the leading suppliers of innovative electrical and digital networked building management systems. The family-owned company, which was founded in 1905, has helped shape the world of electrical systems and intelligent building management with numerous own developments. Innovations such as the Gira HomeServer have helped Gira become a leading pioneer in the development of "Smart Building Systems" and the digitisation of buildings. Gira products and solutions stand for German engineering expertise, reliable "Made in Germany" quality, sustainable production processes, environmentally-friendly and resource-efficient operations and perfect form and function. Most importantly, however, they make people's lives more comfortable, easier and safer. That applies especially to Gira's range of assistance products such as automatic night-lighting systems that provide orientation and safety when visiting the bathroom, or call systems for quickly and easily calling for help in the event of an emergency. It's no coincidence that Gira Assistance products are now used in numerous hospitals and healthcare facilities around the world – for example in the Senior Residence in Erding, in Esslingen Hospice or in the Isala Clinic in Zwolle in Holland. Gira Assistance systems are also used in the public areas of Hamburg's new Elbe Philharmonic Hall. Thanks to its extensive expertise in the field of plastics, Gira has also become a manufacturer of complex plastic products for the medical industry.

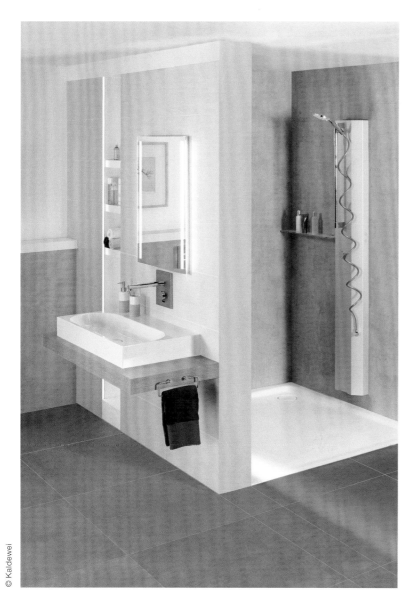

© Kaldewei

KALDEWEI

A perfect match for hospital environments – shower floors and washbasins made of steel enamel

Kaldewei steel enamel – hygienic, safe and cost-effective

Hospital managers face the challenging task of reconciling the need for excellent hygiene with economic considerations. Kaldewei offers a range of solutions specially tailored to the needs of hospitals and healthcare environments: enamel shower surfaces and washbasins made of Kaldewei steel enamel exhibit excellent material properties, guaranteeing not only hygiene and safety in patient bathrooms but also maximum durability and cost-effectiveness.

Kaldewei's SECURE PLUS anti-slip surface finish has been certified by TÜV Rheinland as being compliant with quality class B for wet barefoot areas (DIN 51097) and quality class R10 for anti-slip characteristics in work spaces and working areas with an increased slip risk (DIN 51130).

Every minute counts – easy-clean products

Floor-level shower surfaces by Kaldewei have a hard-wearing enamel surface that is robust and easy to clean, making them ideal for the particular hygiene requirements of hospitals and healthcare facilities. Kaldewei steel enamel is acid and chemical resistant and, therefore, unaffected by medicinal bath additives and disinfectants commonly used in hospitals.

A perfect partner for patient bathrooms

Floor-level shower surfaces and washbasins made of Kaldewei steel enamel offer patient bathrooms uncompromising hygiene paired with elegant design, excellent comfort and anti-slip surfaces for added safety. Kaldewei steel enamel products are ideally suited to the demanding requirements of hospital use, providing a lasting solution that pays off within a short space of time. With a 30-year guarantee that additionally vouches for its quality, Kaldewei is the ideal partner for hospitals and healthcare facilities.

Contact details:
Franz Kaldewei GmbH & Co. KG
Beckumer Str. 33 -35

D-59229 Ahlen
+49 2382 785-0
www.kaldewei.com

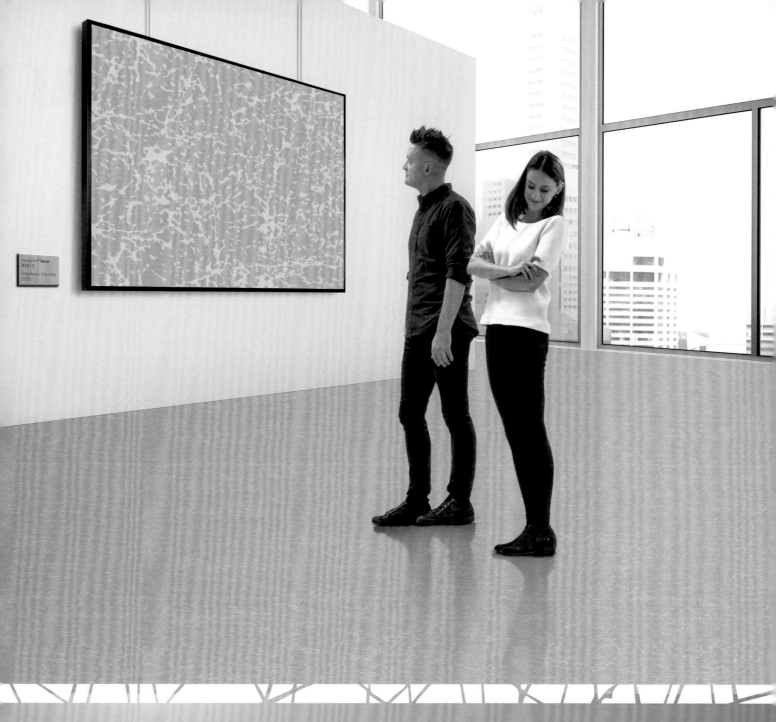

noraplan® lona

IMAGINE YOUR FLOOR AS A WORK OF ART.

The floor as a canvas: noraplan® lona rubber flooring offers a world of new creative possibilities thanks to the state-of-the-art manufacturing technology. Its seemingly random patterns of fine splashes and droplets are inspired by abstract painting techniques. The balance between expressive patterning and pleasing colour blends gives interiors an uplifting, harmonious atmosphere. With excellent hygienic qualities, durable ergonomics and certified environmentally-friendly properties, noraplan® lona is the perfect choice for healing environments.

Be inspired/lch inspirieren:
www.lona.nora.com/lona-en

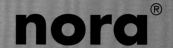

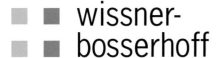

wissner-bosserhoff

Member of LINET Group

Trends in design and functionality

wissner-bosserhoff sees itself as a trendsetter in design and functionality. The beds of the company which belongs to the LINET Group have recently won not only numerous design awards, but also set new standards with their innovative features — in the sense of a European market leader...

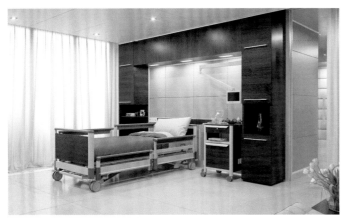

Elegant hotel design for universal and optional service stations

With the image 3 series, wissner-bosserhoff has recently laid an unprecedented success story and more than quintupled the sales figures for hotel hospital beds in the German market. Its balanced relationship of timeless, aluminum-embossed look and homely trend decorations creates a modern look and provides an active healing environment.

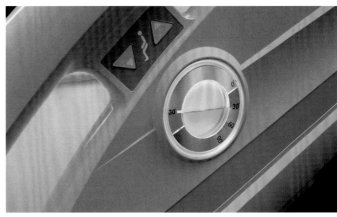

eleganza 2 – New standard for acute care

The eleganza 2 impresses with its uncompromising clinical design, a well thought-out side-rail concept for mobilisation, a multifunctional care system as well as a hygienic and easy-to-clean material mix. Features such as the integrated Mobi-Lift and the integrated angle and altimeter make eleganza 2 unique. It is also universally applicable on all stations.

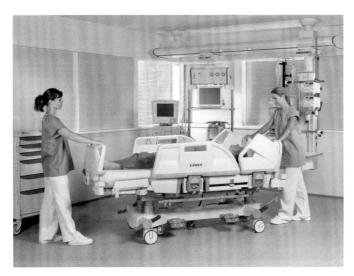

multicare – The intensive bed of the top class

The state-of-the-art intensive care bed multicare relieves the nurses and the patient thanks to reliable high-tech functions in all areas of intensive care. Top features such as the automatic lateral therapy, the high X-ray and C-arm compatibility, an integrated weighing system as well as the electromotoric i-drive for the stress-relieving transport of the bed make multicare the indispensable partner of the patient and intensive care personal.

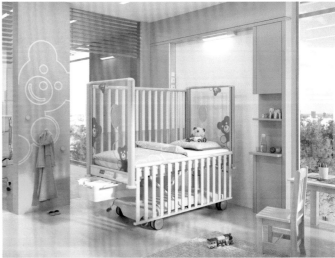

tom 2 – Fully electrically adjustable childrens bed with 360° protection

Modern child beds for patients in preschool age must be safe and also be easily accessible to the nursing staff. The electrically adjustable tom 2 is characterised by a child-friendly and state-of-the-art design with fresh colors. It has been developed in close collaboration with leading European university hospitals and is suitable for all pediatric areas, including intensive care.